Postponing Heaven

groundwork
STUDIES IN THEORY AND SCRIPTURE

The GROUNDWORK series places Mormon scripture in dialogue with contemporary theory. By drawing on a broad range of academic disciplines—including philosophy, theology, literary theory, political theory, social theory, economics, and anthropology—GROUNDWORK books test both the richness of scripture as grounds for contemporary thought and the relevance of theory to the task of reading scripture.

Series Editors

Adam S. Miller
Joseph M. Spencer

Postponing Heaven

The Three Nephites, the Bodhisattva, and the Mahdi

Jad Hatem

Translated by Jonathon Penny

NEAL A. MAXWELL INSTITUTE *for* RELIGIOUS SCHOLARSHIP
Brigham Young University
Provo, Utah

A Groundwork book.

Originally published as *Les Trois Néphites, le Bodhisattva et le Mahdî: Ou l'ajournement de la béatitude comme acte messianique,* Éditions du Cygne, Paris, France, 2007.

Library of Congress Cataloging-in-Publication Data

Names: Hatem, Jad, author. | Penny, Jonathon, translator.
Title: Postponing heaven : the three Nephites, the Bodhisattva, and the Mahdi / Jad Hatem; translated by Jonathon Penny.
Other titles: Trois Néphites, le Bodhisattva et le Mahdî, ou l'ajournement de la béatitude comme acte messianique. English
Description: Provo, Utah : Neal A. Maxwell Institute for Religious Scholarship, Brigham Young University, [2015] | ?2015 | Series: Groundwork : studies in theory and Scripture | Includes index. | Translation of: Les Trois Néphites, le Bodhisattva et le Mahdî, ou l'ajournement de la béatitude comme acte messianique.
Identifiers: LCCN 2015032489 | ISBN 9780842528672 (trade paper : alk. paper) | ISBN 9780842529532 (e pub) | ISBN 9780842529549 (kindle)
Subjects: LCSH: Messianism. | Immortalism. | Nephites. | Bodhisattvas. | Mahdi.
Classification: LCC BL475 .H3813 2015 | DDC 206/.1--dc23
LC record available at http://lccn.loc.gov/2015032489

The paper used in this publication meets the minimum requirements of the American National Standard for Information Sciences—Permanence of Paper for Printed Library Materials. ANSI Z39.48-19

ISBN 978-0-8425-2867-2

Cover design: Ben Dougal

Printed in the United States of America

http://maxwellinstitute.byu.edu

for Karim Assouad

The gods asked me for my
eternal soul
as if it were a spring of gold that
would well up in them.

– Marguerite Yourcenar

Contents

Foreword

AT THE END OF AUGUST 2007, I attended a conference in Sibiu, Romania, entitled "Religious Metaphors and Philosophical Concepts." The conference was followed by a one-week summer course on the same topic at the Bancoveanu Monastery in Romania's Fagaras Mountains. The topic was good. The presenters were excellent, including John Milbank (University of Nottingham) and Jean-Yves Lacoste (Cambridge University). There was also someone I'd not heard of before, Jad Hatem (St. Joseph's University, Beirut).

After two good days in Sibiu, a young and earnest graduate student (Paul Terec) drove me down the bumpy road to the monastery in his own car. On arriving, I settled in and then went for the first night's dinner in the refectory. The entrance was narrow, requiring us to line up to pass through it, and as we were in line I heard someone behind me talking about Mormons. I couldn't hear what the person behind me was saying, but I heard the word *Mormons* several times and began to anticipate a problem, at least a tense moment when it became clear that I am a Latter-day Saint. I'm not naturally paranoid, but my experience with other academics concerning Mormonism has infrequently begun with them thinking good of it.

Entering the refectory, we lined up on two sides of long tables butted end to end, and when I came to my place, I found myself directly opposite the person whom I'd heard speaking. "Oh well," I thought. "I might as well deal with this at the beginning." We then went around the tables, each person introducing himself. When I did so and said, "I'm from Brigham Young University," the fellow across the table from me stood up, reached across to hug me, and said, "BYU! I *love* Mormons!"

Needless to say, I was surprised. I hadn't expected overt hostility, but I'd expected *that* response perhaps even less.

The person who had welcomed me so enthusiastically was Professor Jad Hatem. We talked over dinner and afterward, and as we talked he told me of a book that he had recently published, *Les Trois Néphites, le Bodhisattva et le Mahdî* (Éditions du Cygne, 2007). That is what he had been talking about behind me in line. It was difficult for me to believe that a philosopher from Lebanon had heard enough about Mormons to write about us at all, much less to write about a topic like the Three Nephites.

In the Book of Mormon three of Jesus's disciples in the ancient Americas desire to remain on the earth so that, as Jesus says to them, "ye might bring the souls of men unto me, while the world shall stand" (3 Nephi 28:9). He grants them that blessing:

> Ye shall never taste of death; but ye shall live to behold all the doings of the Father unto the children of men, even until all things shall be fulfilled according to the will of the Father, when I shall come in my glory with the powers of heaven. And ye shall never endure the pains of death; but when I shall come in my glory ye shall be changed in the twinkling of an eye from mortality to immortality; and then shall ye be blessed in the kingdom of my Father. And again, ye shall not have pain while ye shall dwell in the flesh, neither sorrow save it be for the sins of the world; and all this will I do because of the thing which ye have desired of me. (3 Nephi 28:7–9)

Most academic discussions of the Three Nephites investigate their appearances in American folklore, stories of strangers who appear from nowhere to help those in need. Sometimes they change a flat tire. Sometimes they deliver food. They often appear as hitchhikers. And as soon as they've done their good deed, they disappear. That folklore goes significantly beyond the promised blessing in the scriptural text. Needless to say, Jesus says nothing to the three disciples about such things as fixing flat tires. Instead he says they will work to bring souls to Christ, though who would deny that ordinary good deeds are a large part of bringing souls to Christ? The folklore focuses on doing good deeds more than on conversion, and the folklore is what most people, academic or not, probably think of when they think of the Three Nephites.

But Hatem said he had made a philosophical and theological analysis of the relevant verses in the Book of Mormon rather than an analysis of folkloric stories about the Three Nephites. After dinner he gave me a copy of his little volume, and the combination of jet lag and curiosity—and the need to refer often to my French dictionary—kept me up until breakfast the next morning. As a result, I wasn't much good during the next day's lectures, but I was excited by Hatem's book.

Hatem has read the Book of Mormon carefully. He has understood it, and though he sometimes understands things differently than we would—he is, after all, not a Mormon—he has understood Mormonism, and he has offered an original analysis of the passage in 3 Nephi. His argument is that we should understand the Three Nephites as people who, like the bodhisattva in the Buddhist traditions and the Mahdi in Islam, sacrifice their existence not by dying but by consecrating their existence to others. Whereas Christ died for others, making it possible to return to the Father, the Three Nephites are preserved to bring the rest of humanity to him. Mormonism, therefore, understands Christian life as an imitation of the Three Nephites, even if only implicitly.

Like several recent publications, but published in the original before most of them, Hatem's work shows that serious academic reflection is an appropriate response to the Book of Mormon. Of course, reflection on Latter-day Saint theology by non–Latter-day Saints will sometimes disagree with what Latter-day Saints would say. And of course academic reflection is not necessary for Mormon believers or essential to The Church of Jesus Christ of Latter-day Saints. The simplicity of the gospel does not demand philosophical or theological reflection. It requires the simplicity of faith in Jesus Christ and a change of heart that emanates in a new life. But the Neal A. Maxwell Institute is dedicated to the assumption that there is a place for academic reflection on LDS scripture and belief by both Latter-day Saints and non–Latter-day Saints. So the appearance of Hatem's book as the first volume in a series from the Institute dedicated to the rigors of theory and the riches of scripture is entirely appropriate.

By analyzing the story of the Three Nephites, and especially by comparing it to similar beliefs in Buddhism and Islam, Jad Hatem shows us one way of thinking about the Book of Mormon: it has a profound ethical and soteriological teaching about the necessity of self-sacrifice. Hatem's approach is original, especially in that it focuses on a story that many Mormons consider marginal to the book's message. He makes the case that the brief story is emblematic of that message. For me, Hatem turned the Book of Mormon account of the Three Nephites from something that I paid little attention to into a central metaphor for Christian life.

Readers will not find this book light reading. It engages contemporary academic theological and philosophical thought in its own terms. It looks at Mormonism from a non–Latter-day Saint point of view. It is a comparative work as well as a careful reflection on the Three Nephites, so it discusses beliefs of religions with which many English speakers may be unfamiliar. Hatem thinks broadly and creatively, comparing and commenting on religions and literatures. So Hatem's argument takes us along a path to which we must pay attention because, along the way of that path, he takes philosophical and theological excursions. If we confuse the excursions with the path, we will have difficulty understanding what he is saying. This is a style of writing to which most Americans are not accustomed.

This book was written in French by a Lebanese Maronite Catholic. Different language groups and cultures have different styles of writing, so *Postponing Heaven* is an intersection of several different styles: contemporary French philosophy and Maronite Catholic experience among them. The fact that it is a translation into English further complicates matters. So readers will find that this book is written in a style foreign to those accustomed to Anglophonic rhetoric. Such things may be hurdles for readers, but they are not insurmountable. In the end, the argument of *Postponing Heaven: The Three Nephites, the Bodhisattva, and the Mahdi* is well worth the slow and reflective reading that it will require. In places its writing is beautiful. Throughout, its ideas are as well.

James E. Faulconer

Translator's Preface

I do not wish to embellish the borders of this remarkable little book with impertinent observations about my own modest part in making it over for an English-reading audience. In that spirit, I will let the occasional translator's note attend to the occasional snip or snare, and here indulge only in a brief comment about the overall work of translation that has been my privilege.

Translation is, of course, an act of both imitation and interpretation. Done well, it is at once artful and scholarly, but it is most of all an act of faith. A translator has to be faithful to both the style and substance of the original work. But faithfulness to the source is compounded with a second fidelity to the reader's ear and thus to the reader's tongue. Translation is a reworking of the original in new and often stubborn cloth.

Hatem's style is rich, deep, unself-conscious, variously inflected with the playfulness of Continental thought and a further playfulness all his own, and is therefore highly and pleasingly personal. Some of the play—rhythmic, alliterative, allusive—resists translation, threatening garishness or stiffness in coming over, such that the dual fidelities of translation require turning out certain complex phrases in homelier English cloth, and other, plainer phrases spun in muslin, chintz, or *mukayyar*. At times, fidelity requires loosening a knot or two, and at others, tying off errant strands. But on balance, the voice you read in this book is Hatem's, unaccented.

The material is similarly complex and rich, and Hatem's knowledge of the traditions he interrogates is extensive, expert, and easy. Stepping back now and then from some very spirited sentences, I have been impressed by the beauty and sympathy with which he treats the figures—human, messianic, and divine—that populate the work, and the systems of belief in which they operate. He is respectful and clear-sighted, fascinating because he is fascinated by it all himself. His intersection of just these traditions and just these figures in just these ways is compelling and unique, and I predict its lasting place in religious scholarship.

The book is his, but insofar as I have been privileged to help bring it to a broader audience, my own thanks go to many at Salt Press, who set the project going, and at the Maxwell Institute, whose work it has become. But thanks especially to Joseph Spencer and James Faulconer, without whose efforts and expertise the translation would be little more than an amateur effort. And thanks, of course, to Jad Hatem for his patience and for allowing me the privilege of worrying the fabric of his thought in fits and starts for so long. I hope he, and you, will like the cut and carriage of it.

Jonathon Penny, PhD

Introduction

> And if thou draw out thy soul to the hungry, and satisfy the afflicted soul; then shall thy light rise in obscurity, and thy darkness be as the noonday. (Isaiah 58:10)

I SPEAK HERE OF "HUMAN MESSIANICITY," by which I mean the disposition to desire to save others. As an "existential," in other words as belonging to the general theoretical structure of human being prior to any voluntary personal decision, human messianicity is part of the ethical constitution of human being and therefore finds expression in both ordinary and exceptional situations.[1] Messianicity is an acute form of human virtue—the *jen* of the Confucian school radicalized by Mencius, who said that "every man is given a heart that cannot bear the suffering of others. . . . It would be inhuman not to feel compassion."[2] Knowing how to enlarge the compassion we feel for those we perceive to include compassion for those we cannot perceive—achieving universality of compassion—is everything. In Chinese, the logogram *jen* (仁,

1. I have developed this concept of messianicity (messianité) in two French-language publications: Jad Hatem, *Semer le Messie selon Fondane poète* [Sowing the Messiah: The poetry of Fondane] (Brussels: La Part de l'oeil, 2004); and Jad Hatem, *Théologie de l'oeuvre d'art mystique et messianique: Thérèse d'Avila, Andreï Rublev, Michel Henry* [The mystical and messianic work of art: Theresa of Ávila, Andrei Rublev, Michel Henry] (Brussels: Lessius, 2006), particularly chapter 1, section 3. The aim of this book is not to insist on divine or hierarchical messianicity—rather it is, in part, to establish an anthropological basis for divine messianicity (without which Christology would be unthinkable) and more especially to attend to human messianicity, its understudied corollary.

2. *Mencius* II.A.6. The translation used here is *Mencius*, trans. D. C. Lau (New York: Penguin, 2003), 38. *Jen*, which can be translated as "goodness" or "goodwill," is defined by Cheng Yi as the impartiality that puts itself in the shoes of others.

pronounced "ren") embodies this idea since it is composed of both the character for "man" (人) and the figure for "two" (二): *jen* is grounded in simply *being-with*.

It seems right to see this messianic ethic as one of two sources of religion (the other being the mystical). But it is not always easy to locate the messianic core in a religious tradition. In some religions, the deposit is rather meager. In most, it is veiled by a movement of mercy that leads to Incarnation: a divine messianicity. *Human* messianicity is, therefore, all the more precious when we find it unalloyed with the divine. Properly understood, Christianity commingles both.[3]

I intend to place this existential, human messianicity in relation with a desire [*vœu*][4] for longevity of earthly life. Messianicity is challenged by this desire in every soul, which more often than not overshadows the desire to help others. The desire to perpetuate one's life might manifest as egoism, as in Honoré de Balzac's *The Elixir of Life*, or more plainly as a fear of death, as in Simone de Beauvoir's *All Men Are Mortal*. Either way, it is helpful to recall the contempt in which such projects are sometimes held: if successful, they can feel like a curse; gaining life can feel like losing death. This is the fate of the Wandering Jew, a ragged phantom of time, condemned both to die with the last man and, according to Klingemann, to "neither hate nor love anyone."[5]

---

3. In a Feuerbachian approach, one would expect to find only human messianicity, merely projected on the divine. Besides being reductive, this approach does not explain how in the person of Christ both the human and divine intersect.

4. Translator's note: Hatem's *vœu* can mean both "vow" and "wish." His use of the term throughout the book seems to embrace both senses severally and implies other, dimensionally related notions: longing, desire, oath, covenant, invocation, and prayer. "Wish" extends the concept of desire—desire to live in order to serve—and "vow" informs the sacramental and covenantal nature of that life once granted or achieved. The earnestness of the wish and its sacramental nature together suggest the word *prayer*. For the purposes of lexical clarity, where I have translated the word as something other than "vow" according to context, I have inserted "[*vœu*]" to anchor the text to Hatem's central conceit. I should also note that *vœu* more consistently conveys the promissory force of a "vow" as the first chapter develops.

5. Ernst A. F. Klingemann, *Ahasver* (Brunswick: Meyer, 1827), 122.

Despair threatens every effort at saving others bereft of a divine mandate (a mission formally conferred) or of a metaphysical guarantee (the assurance of nirvana), for without at least one of these, success is uncertain. The setbacks typical of a path lined with traps and betrayals may weary and ultimately tempt the sojourner to abandon the path.

Notably, the proposed paradigm for thinking messianicity does not include those who have endowed *themselves* with prolonged life (as opposed to those who receive it as a gift)—even if, as in Taoism, they have healed the sick through spiritual concentration or meditation[6]—for the very good reason that they have not done so *with the aim* of succoring the creatures they heal. Indeed, as in the celebrated case of Lu Tong-Pin, they have only performed good works as a requirement for achieving the immortality they covet for themselves: compassion is just a *means* for them. For the human messiah, blessing others is the *end*.[7]

These preliminary considerations sketch the concepts most salient to the central preoccupation of this book: a *human* messianicity that obtains an indefinite extension of life, but that does so within a *religious* framework. The approach is comparative in order to underline the specific character and conditions of this preoccupation and to bring its implications into full flower. Three particular types are examined: (1) the saved, who resolve to serve humankind (exemplified by the Three Nephites); (2) the self-awakened, who boldly and with resolute heart consecrate themselves to the liberation of other creatures (the bodhisattva); and (3) the righteous, responsible for the world and the establishment of the reign of justice (the Mahdi). Accordingly, the book primarily examines Mormonism, Mahāyāna or "Great Vehicle" Buddhism, and Twelver Shiʿism.

---

6. Cf. *The Book of Chuang Tzu*, chapter 1.

7. The *T'ai-Shang Kan-Ying P'ien* (*The Treatise on the Response of the Tao*) tells us that "in order to be immortalized in heaven, one must perform one thousand, three hundred good deeds; to be immortalized on earth requires three hundred such." Translated from the French rendering by A. Remusat (Paris: Geuthner, 1939), 68. This is just one recipe among many others: taking potions, drugs, and cinnabar; scaling this or that holy mountain; and even, as in the case of the woman Ho Sien-Kou, receiving into oneself the sperm of an immortal will also do nicely.

1

The Vow

The Three Nephites

The Book of Mormon reports the particulars of Christ's post-resurrection ministry to the Nephites, an Israelite people established on the American continent centuries before, at which time Christ chooses from among them twelve disciples. Toward the end of his New World ministry, Christ addresses a question to these Nephite Twelve:

> And it came to pass when Jesus had said these words, he spake unto his disciples, one by one, saying unto them: What is it that ye desire of me, after that I am gone to the Father? And they all spake, save it were three, saying: We desire that after we have lived unto the age of man, that our ministry, wherein thou hast called us, may have an end, that we may speedily come unto thee in thy kingdom. And he said unto them: Blessed are ye because ye desired this thing of me; therefore, after that ye are seventy and two years old ye shall come unto me in my kingdom; and with me ye shall find rest. (3 Nephi 28:1–3)

The desire expressed by these nine disciples is neither astonishing nor very different from the request the mother of James and John makes in the New Testament, which appeal offends the other ten apostles: that her sons take their places in the heavenly kingdom at the right and left hands of Jesus (Matthew 20:21, 24).

The Book of Mormon text continues:

> And when he had spoken unto them [the nine], he turned himself unto the three, and said unto them: What will ye that I should do unto you, when I am gone unto the Father? And they sorrowed in their hearts, for they durst not speak unto him the thing which they desired.
>
> And he said unto them: Behold, I know your thoughts, and ye have desired the thing which John, my beloved, who was with me in my ministry, before that I was lifted up by the Jews, desired of me. Therefore, more blessed are ye, for ye shall never taste of death; but ye shall live to behold all the doings of the Father unto the children of men, even until all things shall be fulfilled, according to the will of the Father, when I shall come in my glory with the powers of heaven. And ye shall never endure the pains of death; but when I shall come in my glory ye shall be changed in the twinkling of an eye from mortality to immortality; and then shall ye be blessed in the kingdom of my Father.
>
> And again, ye shall not have pain while ye shall dwell in the flesh, neither sorrow save it be for the sins of the world; and all this will I do because of the thing which ye have desired of me, for ye have desired that ye might bring the souls of men unto me, while the world shall stand. And for this cause ye shall have fulness of joy; and ye shall sit down in the kingdom of my Father; yea, your joy shall be full, even as the Father hath given me fulness of joy; and ye shall be even as I am, and I am even as the Father; and the Father and I are one. (3 Nephi 28:4–10)

This episode clearly alludes to the biblical pericope where Peter, asking the resurrected Lord what would become of the beloved disciple (whom, for convenience, I will call John), receives the answer: "If I will that he tarry till I come, what is that to thee?" (John 21:22). The brethren take Jesus's response as a promise of immortality, but what follows in the text contradicts such a reading: "Yet Jesus said not unto him, He shall not die; but, If I will that he tarry till I come, what is that to thee?" (John

21:23). The text does not predict that the apostle in question would live an abnormally long life, but rather that Christ would return within the span of a human life.[1] This simple echo of a pronouncement of Jesus reported by the synoptics—"There be some of them that stand here, which shall not taste of death, till they have seen the kingdom of God come with power" (Mark 9:1)—sets John apart and preserves him from martyrdom so that he would survive to see Christ's return.[2] Christ did not return within a generation, however, and John was interred at Ephesus. A certain legend resolves the apparent contradictions: John, Christ's Minister of the Word, merely sleeps while he waits for the Day of the Lord.[3]

The Book of Mormon bears witness of John's longevity in its own way. Does this suggest that its author did not want to take into account the denial recorded in the Gospel of John? Let us say rather that he inscribed his account with a new sense of the nearness of the Lord's coming, one that took shape after the parousia had been deferred and that lends its name to the community founded by Joseph Smith: the Church of Jesus Christ of *Latter-day* Saints. As the risen Christ did not come again in the first centuries of the Christian era, John's longevity necessarily became extraordinary. To reconcile this new order of things with the text of the Gospel, Joseph Smith needed only to invoke an inspired "translation" of the verses. We know that the Pearl of Great Price, part of the canon of Mormon scripture, includes liberal adaptations of Genesis and Matthew, intending to restore their exact meanings, to reveal their cores, and to wipe away the supposed improvements and

1. For a number of exegetes, a certain instability in the formulation of these verses leaves one to think that their redactor seems to refute the implication of immortality for the beloved disciple or to justify his death, which occurred before the glorious return of Christ.

2. The Three Nephites evidently renounce the glory of martyrdom.

3. This is a late tradition known by Augustine. See his *Tractates on the Gospel of John*, 124.22.

inevitable errors of the copyists.[4] Smith undertook such a revision of the Gospel of John as well.[5]

But we have at our disposal a document much more prestigious than a revision, however inspired, of the Johannine verses. In this document, instead of Peter soliciting the Lord for information about John's blessing, John himself pleads with Christ to let him live until Christ returns, not as a witness of his own election, but as a sacrifice permitting him to tirelessly spread the good news and to serve, without ceasing, his fellow beings. The autobiography of Joseph Smith reproduces the text of a revelation given him in April 1829 concerning the question of the beloved disciple's survival. Remarkably, this document (another *Apocryphon of John*?) is supposed to have been written by the beloved disciple himself and then concealed in order to be brought to light much later, in much the same way as the Book of Mormon. Here is the text:

> And the Lord said unto me: John, my beloved, what desirest thou? For if you shall ask what you will, it shall be granted unto you. And I said unto him: Lord, give unto me power over death, that I may live and bring souls unto thee. And the Lord said unto me: Verily, verily, I say unto thee, because thou desirest this thou shalt tarry until I come in my glory, and shalt prophesy before nations, kindreds, tongues and people.

---

4. Although the Bible is included by the Church of Jesus Christ of Latter-day Saints in its corpus of canonical scripture, Mormons, like their founder, consider the Book of Mormon to be "the most correct of any book on earth, and the keystone of our religion." See Joseph Smith Jr., *History of the Church of Jesus Christ of Latter-day Saints*, ed. B. H. Roberts, 7 vols., 2nd ed. (Salt Lake City: Deseret Book, 1978), 4:461; Scott G. Kenney, ed., *Wilford Woodruff's Journal, 1833–1898, Typescript* (Midvale, UT: Signature Books, 1983), 2:139 (November 28, 1841).

5. Smith's description of "translating St. John's Gospel" is found in the heading of Doctrine and Covenants, section 76, which was adapted from "History of the Church" (manuscript), book A-1, p. 183, Church Archives, The Church of Jesus Christ of Latter-day Saints, Salt Lake City, Utah. For Smith's revision of John, see Scott H. Faulring, Kent P. Jackson, and Robert J. Matthews, eds., *Joseph Smith's New Translation of the Bible: Original Manuscripts* (Provo, UT: Religious Studies Center, Brigham Young University, 2004), 442–67.

> And for this cause the Lord said unto Peter: If I will that he tarry till I come, what is that to thee? For he desired of me that he might bring souls unto me, but thou desiredst that thou mightest speedily come unto me in my kingdom. I say unto thee, Peter, this was a good desire; but my beloved has desired that he might do more, or a greater work yet among men than what he has before done. Yea, he has undertaken a greater work; therefore I will make him as flaming fire and a ministering angel; he shall minister for those who shall be heirs of salvation who dwell on the earth. And I will make thee to minister for him and for thy[6] brother James; and unto you three I will give this power and the keys of this ministry until I come. Verily I say unto you, ye shall both have according to your desires, for ye both joy in that which ye have desired. (D&C 7:1–8)

Here it is John, in person, who takes it upon himself to correct the verses of the Gospel that bears his name.

The date of the revelation is not insignificant. This was the month Joseph Smith began to dictate the translation of the Book of Mormon to Oliver Cowdery—whom he had recently met and with whom he would be ordained by Peter, James, and John.[7] The appearance of the idea of the Three Nephites must, therefore, be exactly contemporaneous with the resolution of the Johannine enigma. So it is natural to suppose that the writing of the Book of Mormon began with 3 Nephi, which seems to me the generative starting point of the whole enterprise.

The autobiography indicates that the revelation followed a difference of opinion between Oliver Cowdery and Joseph Smith about how to know whether John was dead or still living. They decided to consult the writings of the apostle. *The History of the Church* does not say

6. This should read "his," unless "brother" can be taken in a larger, moral sense.

7. Oliver Cowdery briefly described the translation of the Book of Mormon and the appearance of the Jewish apostles Peter, James, and John in a series of letters intended to be published in the *Messenger and Advocate* between 1834 and 1835. See Karen Lynn Davidson, David J. Whittaker, Mark Ashurst-McGee, and Richard L. Jensen, eds., *Histories, Volume 1: Joseph Smith Histories, 1832–1844* (Salt Lake City: Church Historian's Press, 2012), 38–44. See also Doctrine and Covenants 27:12–13.

which of them held which hypothesis, but I do not doubt in the least that Joseph was in favor of the miraculous,[8] for it has the virtue both of explaining John's fate as rendered in the Book of Mormon and of throwing a light on the spirit of the Prophet himself: a spirit imbued with messianicity.[9]

I should also note that the two scenes—in which John and the Three Nephites are granted their desires—correspond by design, so much so that John's vow is supposed to have taken place shortly before that of the Three Nephites. This is, among other things, isomorphism, one of the salient traits of the composition of the Book of Mormon, which sees the risen Christ instituting another group of twelve disciples in a new Holy Land.[10]

---

8. There is in the longing of the Three Nephites something like a regulative ideal, so Joseph Smith will not empirically express a desire [*vœu*] for longevity of service, though this will not stop the faithful from believing that he will not taste death: "Some has supposed that Br Joseph Could not die but this is a mistake it is true their has been times when I have had the promise of my life to accomplish such & such things, but having accomplish those things I have not at present any lease of my life I am as liable to die as other men." Andrew F. Ehat and Lyndon W. Cook, eds., *The Words of Joseph Smith: The Contemporary Accounts of the Nauvoo Discourses of the Prophet Joseph* (Provo, UT: Religious Studies Center, Brigham Young University, 1980), 112.

9. To give but one example of messianicity in Joseph's thought: "Love is one of the chief characteristics of Deity, and ought to be manifested by those who aspire to be the sons of God. A man filled with the love of God, is not content with blessing his family alone, but ranges through the whole world, anxious to bless the whole human race." *History of the Church of Jesus Christ of Latter-day Saints*, 4:227; from a letter from Joseph Smith to the Twelve, December 15, 1840, Nauvoo, Illinois, published in *Times and Seasons* (January 1, 1841): 258 (incorrectly dated October 19, 1840, in *History of the Church*).

10. This is not to mention other institutions put in place by Joseph Smith. I should note that the twelve Nephite disciples have an inferior status to that of the twelve Jewish apostles. And it is equally notable that, according to the texts written after the Book of Mormon, God created many worlds (see D&C 76:24; Moses 1:39). If these other worlds are peopled by humans, it is consistent to conclude that at his resurrection, Christ also visited them and instituted other quorums of twelve. The existence of other planets to which "translated" men might be sent in the guise of angels charged with a specific ministry was, in fact, discussed in a sermon given by Joseph in 1840. See Ehat and Cook, *Words of Joseph Smith*, 41.

Another number shows up as well, though slightly altered: three. Although Peter and James did not live excessively long lives, they were charged with assisting John from heaven. This is why they received, with him, a singular priestly consecration—doubtless to the Melchizedek Priesthood—and with it the key of the knowledge of God,[11] which Joseph Smith learned was held by the three apostles (Peter, James, and John)[12] and which they would soon confer on him.[13] Yet if, as Gabriel Marcel profoundly observes, "the most consecrated are the most willing,"[14] the heart of the matter is consecration as such.[15] John's vocation, different as it is from the ministry of the Three Nephites, may well present messianic qualities.

The idea we encounter in the Book of Mormon of postponing the blessings of heaven is all the more worthy of interest for not being drawn from the New Testament, even though Paul, in declaring his desire to be anathema[16] and cut off from Christ if it would bless his people (see Romans 9:3), might be said to reinforce it. That is, although Paul and the Three Nephites share a messianicity ready to renounce

---

11. See Doctrine and Covenants 84:19. Although the Aaronic Priesthood is responsible for the gospel of repentance and baptism (see D&C 13), it has never been "restored" by anyone but Joseph Smith and, strictly speaking, would not have been given to non-Levites in antiquity.

12. The exact date of the conferral of the Melchizedek Priesthood by Peter, James, and John upon Joseph Smith and Oliver Cowdery is not found in the extant sources. See the discussion in *History of the Church*, 1:40–42. The ordination is accounted for in Doctrine and Covenants 27:12. Note that the three Jewish apostles—witnesses to the transfiguration and the resurrection of Jairus's daughter—constitute the intimate circle Jesus invited to Gethsemane.

13. We learn elsewhere that the presiding Twelve of the Church of Jesus Christ of Latter-day Saints hold certain keys exclusively (see D&C 112:15–16).

14. See Gabriel Marcel, *Being and Having*, trans. Katherine Farrer (Westminster: Dacre, 1949), 127, translation modified.

15. Translator's note: Hatem plays on the several meanings of *consécration* and employs Marcel to the same end. The word indicates severally, in order of use, "ordination," "devotion" or "dedication," and "setting apart."

16. That is to say "cut off" or "accursed." In the Septuagint, *anathema* takes the place of the Hebrew *herem*, meaning "destined for total destruction"—destruction that includes erasure from God's memory.

salvation without hesitation, the ways and means diverge. In the first place, the Nephites renounce salvation temporarily. In the second, Paul does not ask for an extension of life because the fulfillment of his desire [*vœu*] would take no more than an instant. Third, out of modesty, the Nephites hardly dare express their desire, whereas the whole force of Paul's desire is in solemn declaration: he would like to win over the Jews by an impetuous love that dares to desire the undesirable. One can also appreciate these nuances by recourse to the distinction between two modes of substitution: one *in the place of others* and one *beneath others.*[17] Paul sees himself in the first of these modes; the Three Nephites see themselves in the second. This same distinction reveals the special messianic features of the permanent ministry of the Three Nephites. Their stewardship is a continual presence of Christ among his people, of solicitude and succor—let us say, of *phoria* (in other words, of bearing and being, as in the root of the words *euphoria* and *dysphoria*).

The Three Nephites are the three mysterious pillars upon which the church is built. Their vocation is not vicarious physical suffering and certainly not vicarious death. But are they, for all that, delivered from every thorn in the flesh? Not if by this we understand something other than bodily pain or natural weakness. Not if by this we understand not only the fatigue occasioned by their apostolic mission—of which Joseph Smith declared that "translation obtains deliverance from the tortures and sufferings of the body but their existence will prolong as to their labors and toils of the ministry before they can enter into so great a rest and glory"[18]—but also affective suffering, for surely they carry a wound: one caused by iniquity. Indeed, it is said, "Therefore, that they might not taste of death there was a change wrought upon their bodies, that they might not suffer pain nor sorrow *save it were for the sins of the world*" (3 Nephi 28:38, emphasis added).

A substantial modification to their metabolism must be imagined in support of Mormon theologian Bruce R. McConkie's thesis that blood

17. Cf. Jad Hatem, *Mystique et philosophie mêlées* [Mysticism and philosophy mingled] (Paris: L'Harmattan, 2005), chapter 1, section 2.

18. Ehat and Cook, *Words of Joseph Smith*, 42.

does not circulate any more in the bodies of "translated" beings who, once translated, may uniquely live within the physical and metaphysical worlds at the same time.[19] This would imply great speed of movement, but not ubiquity of presence. The Three Nephites, having from this point on qualities of the angels, obtain the power to show themselves to anyone they like (3 Nephi 28:30). Let me add that the devil has no power over them, for "there was a change wrought upon them, insomuch that Satan could have no power over them, that he could not tempt them; and they were sanctified in the flesh, that they were holy, and that the powers of the earth could not hold them" (3 Nephi 28:39).

The Mahdi

Under these conditions, the fate of the Three Nephites invites a comparison with that of the Twelfth Imam of Twelver Shiʿism: the Mahdi, son of Hassan al-Askari. Like other immaculate Imams (*maʿsūm*), he is twice mediator, as the face by which Allah is approached,[20] and as the Ark of Salvation,[21] insofar as he derives from the Creator's mercy spread over his creatures.[22] Guided himself,[23] the Mahdi guides his people toward

19. See Bruce R. McConkie, *The Millennial Messiah* (Salt Lake City: Deseret Book, 1982), 644.

20. See Ibn Bābūya, *Kamāl al-dīn wa-tamām al-niʿmah* (Beirut: Al-Aʿlamī, 2004), 222. "He who knows us, knows Allah," the Imams' refrain (ibid., 248, translated from Hatem's rendering in French). Or again: "By our manner of worship Allah is worshiped." Ibn Bābūya, *Kitāb al-tawḥīd* (Tehran: n. p., 1978), 152 (translated from Hatem's rendering in French).

21. In Arabic, the *safinat al-najāt*. See Muhammad ibn Ibrahim al-Nuʿmānī, *Kitāb al-ghaybat* (Qom: n. p., 2005), 37.

22. Ibn Bābūya, *Kamāl al-dīn wa-tamām al-niʿmah*, 198.

23. This is the first sense of the word *Mahdi* and one that applies to all Twelve Imams, but it does not convey the total register of signification in the Arabic word. Changing the voice from passive to active is common, as if *Mahdi* were merely a synonym for *hadi* (guide). It was said of the Fifth Imam, Muhammad al-Bāqir, that "he is called the Mahdi because he will guide us to a hidden reality." Al-Nuʿmānī, *K'itāb al-ghaybat*, 243 (translated from Hatem's rendering in French). For more on the title *hadi*, see ibid., 232.

paradise.[24] Keeper of the initiatory knowledge, he is the exegete par excellence of the divine verses.[25] His presence on the earth is necessary in order to guard against annihilation, because he is the pillar of the world. "The world is never without an Imam, declared one among them, Jaffar al-Saddik, because without him, it would be undone."[26] It is by the Mahdi that Allah keeps the sky from falling to the earth.[27] His absence, even for an hour,[28] even for the blink of an eye,[29] would be catastrophic.

The Mahdi is reminiscent of the Jewish tradition of the thirty-six righteous men—the *Lamed-Vav Tzaddiqim*—by whose merits the world continues to exist.[30] Like the Three Nephites and the Mahdi, the *Tzaddiqim* lead a hidden existence entirely devoted to safeguarding creation. And as with their Mormon and Islamic counterparts, being unknown does not prevent them from radiating light and heat, any more than veiling cloud interrupts the sun.[31] But unlike their counterparts, they

---

24. Ibn Bābūya, *Kamāl al-dīn wa-tamām al-niʿmah*, 198.

25. Among the stories about the Mahdi's important future acts, one point of comparison deserves attention, even though it does not directly address our topic. Following the instructions of the angel Moroni, Joseph Smith purportedly unearthed the Book of Mormon, which had been buried on the American continent in the fifth century after Christ. It is also said that the Mahdi is called by that name because he will be guided (yuhdā) toward a hidden reality and will retrieve the Torah and the Gospels from a land called Antioch (variant: from a mountain in Syria) in order to be able to judge the Jews and the Christians by their own books. See Al-Asfahānī, *Muʿjam al-malāhim wa-l-fitan* (Tehran: n.p., 2002), 1:199. There is an obvious difference here: the Torah and the Gospels the Mahdi discovers are unaltered, familiar texts, whereas according to the angel, the Book of Mormon, said to contain the fulness of the eternal gospel, is obscure. But there is also another similarity: Joseph Smith held that the supreme Father will judge those who possess a law according to the terms of that law, and will judge without recourse to a law those who live without one. See the editorial published in the *Times and Seasons* (April 15, 1842): 759; *History of the Church*, 4:595–96.

26. Quoted in Muhammad Yaʿqūb al-Kulaynī, *Usūl al-kāfī* (Beirut: Dāt al-adwā, 1992), 1:234.

27. Ibn Bābūya, *Kamāl al-dīn wa-tamām al-niʿmah*, 199.

28. Al-Nuʿmānī, *Kitāb al-ghaybat*, 140, 144.

29. Ibn Bābūya, *Kamāl al-dīn wa-tamām al-niʿmah*, 197.

30. See Babylonian Talmud *Sanhedrin* 97ab.

31. This is said of the Mahdi, the hidden Imam, in Muhammad Baqir Majlesi, *Bihār al-Anwār* (Beirut: Al-Wafāʾ, 1983), 52:92–93. Too much sunlight dazzles and

do not enjoy longevity: the Eternal is content to raise up replacements of the same moral quality in perpetuity. Mystical Islam has its own version of the *Tzaddiqim*: the *abdāl*. But Mormonism has no need of such figures, and even among the Shiʿites the tradition of the *abdāl* came to an end with the Twelfth Imam, whose mission will end only with time itself. The first eleven Imams, however, reached the hereafter in succession, as the nine Nephite disciples did (in their case, almost simultaneously).

It is important to note that the indefinite extension of earthly life is not immortality in any strict sense, which is God's prerogative, as the Apostle Paul is wont to underscore (see 1 Timothy 6:16). The Qurʾan proclaims, "Every soul shall taste of death" (3:185; 21:35). Without divine consideration, the Shiʿite Mahdi would be assassinated. He is capable of dying. The same is true of the Three Nephites, who will, Christ promises, put on incorruptibility in the blink of an eye at the time of his Second Coming; although this change is instantaneous, it is a kind of death, for death is inscribed in all flesh (see 2 Nephi 9:4, 6).

The possibility of death is thus constitutive of every human, but this does not mean that every human dies,[32] nor does it stop us from imagining an alternative material transformation, as in the case of the Three Nephites. One tradition relating to the Mahdi holds that he will have the body of a forty-year-old man until his death.[33] Another claims that, like other Imams, he will not cast a shadow.[34] One would rightly reckon that in the way of Adam in Eden, the Mahdi is never ill.[35] But we cannot say, as we can of the Taoist saints, that his existence is nothing but life.[36]

---

inflicts blindness—that is to say, ignorance (see ibid., 94).

32. Or even all humans. Saint Augustine asserts that, during his paradisiacal existence, Adam possessed both mortality (by nature) and immortality (by grace) at once, for "*poterat non mori*"—he could not die. See Augustine, *The Literal Meaning of Genesis* VI.25–26. It was sin that introduced death.

33. See Ibn Bābūya, *Kamāl al-dīn wa-tamām al-niʿmah*, 591.

34. See Shafīq Jarādī, *Rashaḥāt wilāʾīyah* (Beirut: n. p., 2006), 66.

35. See Augustine, *City of God* XIV.26.

36. See Lao Tzu, *Tao Te Ching*, 50.

His condition is distinguishable from that of the thirty-six *tzaddiqim*, who wait for the Messiah's irruption in history, and from the Three Nephites, who attend his glorious return, because in Twelver Shiʿism, the Mahdi is himself the object of eschatological hope. Does he, in some way, control history? In some measure, yes—for if, as Kulaynī reports, the Imams die only when they choose to,[37] the Mahdi could come from among them at the last day to hasten the end of time (the old tradition requires that he live a mere twenty years or so after the establishment of his reign). But since the Mahdi is not Allah himself, he remains subject to a higher jurisdiction, and in this way he resembles the Jewish Messiah.

As to whether or not earthly existence constitutes, in the Mahdi's eyes, a sacrifice, we can only speculate. One Shiʿite tradition asserts that during the battle of Karbalā, which saw the Mahdi's ancestor, Imam Hussein, and almost his entire family massacred, the Imam had to choose between an angelic intervention on his behalf and the final encounter with God.[38] His preference for the latter shows in him the prevalence of the mystical over the ethical; in the Mahdi, however, the contrary pertains: the mystical is subordinate to the ethical.

With this in mind, we ought to distinguish the reasons for his Occultation, or his becoming hidden (the Minor in 874 CE, the Major in 941 CE), from the reasons for the extension of his life. The oldest of his followers, naturally ignorant of this extension, explained the Mahdi's concealment as a result of his fear of being killed,[39] carrying death (as Valéry puts it) as "a secret child already fully formed."[40] Even were the Mahdi to live to a venerable age, his death would be premature (a *mors immatura*).

37. See al-Kulaynī, *Usūl al-Kāfī*, 1:258–60.

38. See ibid., 1:319.

39. Ibid., 1:398–99, 401. Cf. Muḥammad ibn al-Ḥasan Mahdī, *Adʿiyat al-Imām al-Mahdi* (Beirut: Dār al-Murtadā, 2000), 44.

40. *La Jeune Parque*.

But this episode also invokes a test of denial to which Shiʿites were required to submit,[41] which, from the Occultation on, has tended principally to the biblical and cosmic (notably zodiacal) symbolism of the number twelve, revived by a remark attributed to the Prophet Muhammad, in fulfillment of which twelve vicars born to his tribe—the Quraysh—would succeed him.[42] If there could not be a Thirteenth Imam, and if the lightsome Advent were delayed, the Twelfth would have to remain in place as the Proof for God and his justice before the believers and as Living Qur'an among them in order to guide and heal them;[43] to protect and even to embellish their being by his presence;[44] to make ready for the plan, for the moment God has chosen[45] to avenge the Prophet's family of the cruel and immoral humiliations they suffered; and at the end of an eschatological struggle, to fill the world as much with justice as it had been previously filled with iniquity and tyranny.[46] Since human history itself cannot justify terminating the immoral life by constituting a civil society that administers rights universally, it will fall to the Mahdi to

---

41. Cf. Ibn Bābūya, *ʿIlal al-sharāʾiʿ wa-l-ahkām* (Najaf: n.p., 1966), 1:244. See also Abū Jaʿfar al-Tūsī, *Kitāb al-ghaybat* (Beirut: Muassasat dār al-kitāb, 1988), 203 (on the motif of sifting: 206); al-Nuʿmānī, *Kitāb al-ghaybat*, 24, 170, 210–12.

42. Cf. al-Nuʿmānī, *Kitāb al-ghaybat*, 65–104.

43. See Muḥammad Bāqir al-Ṣadr, *Tārīkh al-ghaybah al-sughrá* (Qom: n.p., 2006), 126.

44. For example, in al-Ḥasan Mahdī, *Adʿiyat al-Imām al-Mahdi*, 84.

45. This is an important point. The Mahdi would have said, "There is no Manifestation (*zuhur*, implying his own), without God's authority (or will)." Quoted in Al-Ṣadr, *Tārīkh al-Ghaybah al-Sughrá*, 308. This does not prevent subjective points of view, such as declaring that the Occultation will last as long as the Mahdi is in danger (see ibid., 131).

46. The Mahdi's messianic ethic clearly raises questions of political theology that neither the bodhisattva nor the thirty-six righteous men worry over. Nor does the Book of Mormon develop a political discourse about the Three Nephites, though it could have, conferring on them a specific millennial role, for instance; they will judge Lehi's descendants, but only in quorum with the other nine (see 1 Nephi 12:10; 3 Nephi 27:27; Mormon 3:19) since supreme power will be held by Christ exclusively. The Immortals of Taoism are the most indifferent to political power: even if all of humanity pled with them to govern the world, they would not condescend to burden themselves so, since calamities never reach them! See *The Book of Chuang Tzu*, chapter 1.

impose such a program by means of a violent rupture and by virtue of his incarnating wisdom in the world.

Explanations of the Mahdi's longevity tend to the miraculous. There is another line of reasoning that lists a number of persons whose lives lasted several centuries without necessarily contradicting natural law. Yet Ibn Bābūya—who uncovers a long list of people who attained a very advanced age, emphasizing Noah[47] in an attempt to make the case of the Mahdi banal—overlooks that these people age, which makes them extraordinary in a different way.[48]

Clearly, the Mahdi does not need to wish [*vœu*] for excessive longevity. The situation itself guarantees it to him for as long as he is bound—by election and (pre-existentiell) ontological worthiness—to his mission, which he consecrates for a testimony.[49] The Shiʿites declare that he became Imam at his father's death, when he was not yet ten years old. If this is so, he would have had no time to request longer life, much less acquire merits to use in the service of his community.[50]

---

47. Ibn Bābūya, *Kamāl al-dīn wa-tamām al-niʿmah*, 302, 473, 482. Noah lived for 2,500 years, according to Majlesi, *Bihār al-Anwār*, 52:200.

48. Ibn Bābūya himself sets Khodr aside because he drank the elixir of life. See Ibn Bābūya, *Kamāl al-dīn wa-tamām al-niʿmah*, 362.

49. Translator's note: the term *existentiell* is paired with the term *existential* in Martin Heidegger, *Being and Time*, trans. John Macquarrie and Edward Robinson (New York: Harper and Row, 1962), 33. *Existentiell* means the understanding we have that comes by way of existing, though it is not necessarily a conscious understanding. *Existential* describes what is characteristic of the structure of existence.

50. However, I would tighten up the hypothesis of the vow by default because the possibility of forfeiture cannot be excluded a priori. By virtue of his transcendental liberty, the Mahdi gives his word. If it is true that "being absolutely available to others precludes the right to dispose freely of oneself" and that "suicide is tied to unavailability" (Marcel, *Being and Having*, 124, translation modified), then were he to commit suicide or allow himself to be killed, were he to merely think of it, the era of justice would be so completely undone that humanity would immediately be summoned for the last judgment. He does not need to give his word again because the power of transcendental liberty that he experiences relieves him of the capacity to revoke that word. On this last point, see Karl Rahner, *Foundations of Christian Faith: An Introduction to the Idea of Christianity* (New York: Seabury, 1978), 129.

The Bodhisattva

No, it is rather the Awakened One, the bodhisattva, who worries about acquiring merit, as reported by a seventh-century Mahayanist writer, Šāntideva, in a work of rare density: "Having completed all these rites, and by virtue of the merit I have acquired, may I be for all beings he who soothes their hurts!"[51] In prefacing this vow by recalling his achievements,[52] the bodhisattva enters into a logic of accumulation that will allow him to transfer substantial merit from himself to others: Christ is a storehouse of merit because of the crucifixion; the bodhisattva's value derives from his asceticism and his elevation. But whereas Christ blesses humankind with the merits produced *by* his Passion, the bodhisattva applies the merits earned in service *toward* his own enlightenment. Both exert themselves, but the bodhisattva does so in order to be able to share what he accumulates,[53] the Christ in sharing what he has already won.[54]

From the moment of his conception, Christ lived for others. This is not true of the bodhisattva, who must, first of all, recognize that a return to himself would be feckless: "His benevolence is indefatigable because he perceives the inexistence—the emptiness—of his self."[55] So it is that

---

51. Šāntideva, *Bodhicaryāvatāra* III.7 (translated from the French as quoted by Hatem; see *La Marche à la lumière*, trans. L. Finot [Paris: Bossard, 1920]).

52. The Bhodisattva's six perfections include generosity (notably in his teaching of the law), morality (in both abstention and action), patience (in enduring injury, etc.), energy (which must be inexhaustible in equal measure with the number of creatures in the world), concentration in meditation, and wisdom. Cf. Asaṅga, *Mahāyāna-Sūtra-Saṁgraha* ad. IV.9.

53. "I must acquire numerous virtues, for me and for others." Šāntideva, *Bodhicaryāvatāra* VII.35 (translated from the French as quoted by Hatem).

54. This comparison overlooks the eucharistic dimension of the gift of self, which can be understood as an exertion *by* distribution (and not only exertion *for* distribution), because it is not held in common among churches calling themselves Christian.

55. Translated from Carré's French as quoted by Hatem; see *Soûtra de la Liberté inconcevable: Enseignements de Vimalakîrti*, trans. P. Carré (Paris: Fayard, 2000). For an English source, see *The Holy Teaching of Vimalakīrti: A Mahāyāna Scripture*, trans. Robert A. F. Thurman (University Park: Pennsylvania State University Press, 1976), 57. One may remark an apparent divergence from the position Lévinas maintains in

a *bodhisattva mahasattva* (a great being), the Compassionate One, *Avalokiteśvara* (he who lowers his gaze toward the world), progressively imbued with the aura of legend, begins his career considering as void the five aggregates that make up the phenomenal world: forms, sensations, perceptions, mental productions, and awareness.[56] Since egoism is no longer possible, love becomes allocentric (or "other-centered") and totally disinterested at the same time: "If you do something in the interest of others, there is no room for pride! no room for complacency! no room for retribution! You must have but one passion: a passion for the well-being of others."[57]

No longer possessing a self, the bodhisattva can give away everything he has. And he need not fear death.[58] Drawing heavily on psychological stratagems in establishing a foundation for the principles of emptiness, Śāntideva goes as far as to invite the candidate to universal commiseration, calling compassion the "mother of the health of all men,"[59] to convince the candidate of a shift in the limits of egoity or even a transfer to others of his own ipseity (or "self-identity") in such a way that the concern for others will not run up against a commonplace caring for self:

> Why not consider as "me" the body of others? As to recognizing our own bodies as strangers, this is an accepted idea and presents no difficulty. In considering that one is oneself full of faults and

Otherwise Than Being, that subjectivity consists in vulnerability and exposition to others. True, he thinks subjectivity starting from the desubstantiation of the subject and with substitution. See Emmanuel Lévinas, *Otherwise Than Being, or Beyond Essence*, trans. Alphonso Lingis (Pittsburgh: Duquesne University Press, 1997).

56. From the Heart Sutra.

57. Śāntideva, *Bodhicaryāvatāra* VIII.109 (translated from Finot's French as quoted by Hatem).

58. *The Flower Ornament Scripture* L.10 (translated from Hatem's French rendering). The list of possessions from which he is disposed to give alms is impressive: it includes his wealth, his wife and children, his limbs, head, eyes, etc. (see ibid., I.21).

59. Śāntideva, *Bodhicaryāvatāra* X.13 (translated from Finot's French as quoted by Hatem). Regarding the ten kinds of commiseration, see *Flower Ornament Scripture* III.2.

> that others are oceans of qualities, one will apply oneself to reject one's own personality and adopt that of someone else. One is interested in one's members as parts of one's body, why not in men as parts of humanity? From habit, we apply the idea of me to this body without soul: why not to others? In this way, if we do good to others, we will feel neither pride nor complacency. One does not hope for recompense because one is nourished oneself.[60]

How remarkable the effect of this emptiness! Transfer of merit to others is possible because there is, at bottom, no self. As the ego and its artifices mount real resistance to such emptiness in the world, a coup is necessary: the simple transfer (considering others as myself) is not enough; I must also consider myself a stranger. (Indeed, the bodhisattva counsels his ego to despair of all self-interest because he has sold it to others.)[61] This is a double movement that Šāntideva formulates as the inversion of ego and others.[62] Our reaction to the intolerable envelops the universe and determines the virtue of humanity beyond what Mencius had conceived. What the Chinese sage deems natural—kindness—requires, according to the Indian, transmutation by decentering the person whose soul is engraved with a will to be only toward himself and by reidentifying the self with others. Hence the sage's astonishment at the bodhisattva: "This pearl of beings, this unprecedented pearl: how is it born since none else feels inclination, or interest, in the well-being of others?"[63] Lao-Tzu's astonishment is more pronounced, for he holds that a saint imitates heaven and earth by *not* showing benevolence (*jen*) toward people, whom he considers straw dogs![64] The bodhisattva seemed to him to contradict nature.

---

60. Šāntideva, *Bodhicaryāvatāra* VIII.112–16; cf. VIII.158 (translated from Finot's French as quoted by Hatem).

61. See ibid., VIII.170. The bodhisattva similarly renounces his body, keeping it solely as an instrument of action (ibid., VIII.184).

62. See ibid., VIII.120.

63. Ibid., I.25 (translated from Finot's French as quoted by Hatem).

64. Lao Tzu, *Tao Te Ching*, 5.

In contrast with Christ (whose disposition in favor of the world preceded his Incarnation), awareness comes to the bodhisattva as a result of his awakening. Hence the necessity of a formal engagement that raises *being-for-others* to the level of *being-toward* on the ruins of *being-for-self*:

> May I be the remedy for illness, the doctor, the nurse, until the illness is extinguished! May I allay with showers of food and drink the torments of hunger and thirst, and in times of famine, become myself drink and nourishment. May I be for the poor an inexhaustible treasure, to be ready to render to them the services they desire! All my future incarnations, all my possessions, all my merit past, present, and future—I renounce them with indifference so that the purpose of all beings might be fulfilled. *Nirvana* is to give up all, and my soul aspires to *nirvana*. Since I must renounce all, it is better to give it to others. I deliver this body to the good pleasure of all beings, that without ceasing they beat, violate, and cover it with dust! That they make of my body a toy, an object of derision and amusement! I gave them my body, what does it matter to me? That they make it do whatever they will! So long as I am not the cause for harm to anyone! If their heart is inflamed and malevolent because of me, let this too serve to realize the ends of all! That those who slander me, harm me, mock me, with all the others, obtain *bodhi*! May I be the protector of the abandoned, guide to those who walk the path, and, for those who desire the other shore, may I be the raft, the crossing, the bridge; may I be a light to those who need a light, a bed to those who need a bed, the slave of those who need a slave; may I be the miracle Stone, the Urn abundant, the magic Formula, the plant which heals, the wishing Tree, the Cow of desires! Just as the earth and the other elements serve many purposes for innumerable beings spread wide in infinite space, even so may I be useful in all ways to them that occupy that space, even if they will not be delivered for an age.[65]

---

65. Šāntideva, *Bodhicaryāvatāra* III.8–22 (translated from Finot's French as quoted by Hatem).

This is quite a contrast with the ideal of buddhahood in Hīnayāna (Lesser Vehicle) Buddhism, where the saint, now entered into nirvana, cuts himself off from humanity, having pursued his own salvation exclusively! The bodhisattva slows his own liberation indefinitely by not severing the lines of transmigration. In taking upon himself, by virtue of universal compassion, the ordeals [*calvaires*] of other beings, and in working to instruct and liberate them by means of the merits he has accumulated, he shows that *their* deliverance, not his, is what motivates him.[66] He does not aspire to awakening, does not accumulate virtue, and does not identify himself with the body of wisdom except for the good of others: "For all the good deeds he performs, he expects not the least recompense."[67] He takes the place of others for pure love, not for algophilia, the love of pain in others or himself.

The nature of the bodhisattva's vow implies that he will be the last to enter into nirvana at the very end of all the cycles and all the centuries of time, if that day ever comes. His continual and eternally unchanging presence on the earth (here the equivalent of longevity) is in no way a source of joy, but really a pure and simple calamity freely desired.[68] The remarkable thing about the bodhisattva is that he confers this presence upon himself, which is to say by retrenchment or suspension of extinction (and not by addition and transfiguration as for the Three Nephites). He both makes the vow to live and assures the conditions of its realization because on the one hand there is in Buddhism no instance of a superior personage (God), and on the other Buddhism

66. See Šāntideva, *Šikshā-Samuccaya* XVI.

67. *Holy Teaching of Vimalakīrti*, 36 (translated from Carré's French as quoted by Hatem). This does not constitute a critique of the Buddha, who, identified with the Absolute in Mahāyāna (Great Vehicle) Buddhism, would have needed a mere gesture in order to extinguish his body and enter into nothingness. He would not cease, therefore, to teach the law, and the length of his life is incalculable. Cf. *The Saddharma-Puṇḍarīka* XVI.

68. This calamity would not serve to assure his salvation—this happened to the sinners of ancient times according to the Book of Mormon: "And the days of the children of men were prolonged, according to the will of God, that they might repent while in the flesh" (2 Nephi 2:21).

allows for repeated incarnations until deliverance. This is different from the idea we find in Goethe, where Faust becomes convinced that he is immortal, that Nature will simply replace his present form when it can no longer contain his spirit. Nor is the bodhisattva a *natura naturans* (or "the self-creating activity of nature") like Raphael, who, according to Nietzsche, would never have to die.[69] Rather, the bodhisattva's vow involves a compassion that offers itself, vowing to attend carefully to all creatures and protect them from evil, to obtain for them an outpouring of blessings, and to work to that end endlessly, in things great and infinitely small alike.[70]

This outpouring is not the grace of a God, but a surplus of messianicity via a relation to the fact of natural death as well as to the imperatives of reincarnation, which ensures the bodhisattva's survival. If freedom really is the way of humanity throughout time, an individual only navigates it with a vow. "Only love possesses the talisman of eternal peace," Novalis would say.[71] Like Christ, the bodhisattva is choked by the misery of men because of their sins. In taking the irrevocable decision to be in agony until the very end of the world, in the manner of Pascal's Christ, he allows the idea of a human messianicity to achieve full flower. His life elucidates the affective foundation of human messianicity:

> The bodhisattva has a marrow-deep love for all creatures, like one might have for an only child; his love works endlessly to keep them safe. . . . Like a dove cherishes her little ones, remains with and broods over them, destroying repulsion by this love; so it is with the Compassionate in relation to all creatures, who are his children.[72]

---

69. See Friedrich Nietzsche, *Untimely Meditations*, trans. R. J. Hollingdale (New York: Cambridge University Press, 1997), 100–107 (II, §8).

70. On this last point, see Jad Hatem, *Charité de l'infinitésimal, variations leibniziennes* [Charity of the infinitesimal: Leibnizian variations] (Paris: L'Harmattan), 2007.

71. Jochen Schulte-Sasse et al., ed., *Theory as Practice: A Critical Anthology of Early German Romantic Writings* (Minneapolis: University of Minnesota Press, 1997), 129.

72. Maitreyanātha/Āryāsaṅga, *Mahāyānasūtrālaṁkāra* XIII.20, 22 (translated from S. Lévy's French as quoted by Hatem).

For this reason, the bodhisattva ranks among the mystics of pure love whose worth, in its excess, surpasses all limits. A logic of scale pertains:

> A person who, on occasion and without real regard, makes a meager donation of food to a few of the poor, enough to support them for only half a day, is celebrated as a saint. What to say, then, of him who gives to an infinite number of souls, for time without end, all that they desire, endlessly, until all living beings meet their end.[73]

We can say in the case of the bodhisattva that his love is excessive, but also that his case rests on a sure foundation.

Earlier, I mentioned the notion of *being-toward*. This modality of intersubjectivity acquires, in the context of messianicity, the value of placing the self at the mercy of others. "I belong to others!" the bodhisattva tells himself. "This must be your conviction, oh my heart! Their well-being must be your only concern from now on!"[74] And from this moment, he sees being present to others as the vector of an infinite availability.[75]

Very different is the attenuated modality of the postponement of heaven portrayed by André Schwarz-Bart in *The Last of the Just*. Schwarz-Bart imagines Yeshua (Jesus considered as a righteous Jew, no more and no less) waiting at the gates of paradise so as not to forget humankind in favor of the Messiah, for whom he also waits.[76] The attenuation of this modality is to be found in its inefficacy. While living,

---

73. Šāntideva, *Bodhicaryāvatāra* I.32–33 (translated from Finot's French as quoted by Hatem).

74. Ibid., VIII.137 (translated from Finot's French as quoted by Hatem).

75. One might think once more of Gabriel Marcel: "I belong to you. This means: I am opening an unlimited credit account in your name, you can do what you want with me, I give myself to you. This does not mean, at least not in principle: I am your slave; on the contrary, I freely put myself in your hands; the best use I can make of my freedom is to place it in your hands; it is as though I freely substituted your freedom for my own; or paradoxically, it is by that very substitution that I realize my freedom." Gabriel Marcel, *Creative Fidelity*, trans. Robert Rosthal (New York: Farrar, Straus, 1964), 40.

76. See André Schwarz-Bart, *The Last of the Just*, trans. Stephen Becker (New York: Atheneum, 1961), 319–29.

the just provides the offices of intercession and substitution. In dying, however, he leaves his place to another and no longer carries on his old mission. The Yeshua of the novelist thus does not resemble the bodhisattva, who has dedicated body and soul to all created beings. He is content to be present to them in prayer and deprives himself of paradise only in sympathetic expectation.[77] This is neither preaching nor direct action like that of the bodhisattva, but participation.

In *The Last of the Just*, then, Yeshua's death is taken seriously and, in consequence, so is his suffering, even without the redemptive value assigned to it by Christians. The Muslim tradition, which holds that the Son of Mary eludes the cross that he might be held in reserve for the era of justice, runs counter: *Issa* will descend from one of the heavens at the end of time,[78] either as the Mahdi (as most Sunnis contend)[79] or as a stand-in for the Twelfth Imam (according to the Shiʿites). Like the novelist's Yeshua, he is both absent from the world in the flesh and yet present to it—more so because, being yet alive, he is able to return. This characterization makes him susceptible, in the popular (and novelistic) imagination, to combination with other forms, like one sees in Orhan Pamuk:

> Liberation might be just around the corner; at our darkest hour, someone might emerge to deliver us from wretchedness. A savior who's walked this earth before, perhaps centuries before, will come back to life as someone else; five hundred years after his death,

---

77. For an idea of what Yeshua deprives himself of, see (among other delights) in the Talmud at the Taanit treatise (31a), which imagines that the Eternal will organize a dance for the just in paradise and that he will count himself among them. See Michael L. Rodkinson, ed., *Babylonian Talmud: Taanit* 31a.

78. The pilgrims of the ascension will meet him in the second heaven, according to Ibn ʿArabi, *The Meccan Revelations*, 2 vols., trans. William C. Chittick, James W. Morris, Cyrille Chodkiewicz, and Denis Gril (New York: Pir, 2002–2004).

79. In a remark attributed to him by the Sunnis, Muhammad announces, "There is no Mahdi but Jesus, son of Mary." Muslim Ibn al-Hajjaj, *Ṣaḥiḥ* (Cairo: n.p., 1873), 2:304.

> He'll come back to Istanbul as Mevlana Celâlettin or Sheikh Galip or perhaps even a newspaper columnist![80]

It is not clear if this passage deals with a resurrection from the dead (which would lend itself to the change in his appearance) or a period of latency, or more simply a lifting up (the title of *qā'im*—Resurrector—being assumed by the Shiʿite Mahdi,[81] he who had never been to hades). What is clear is this: Pamuk conceives a discontinuity by which the ravages that envelop the world may be explained.

There is, finally, a messianic vow that does not require a prolonged mortality but does require a renouncement of paradise: the desire that heaven give way to earth. True, the labor this entails precludes the possibility of experiencing supreme pleasure. And one is right to ask if this vow, expressed so poignantly by Thérèse de Lisieux as she neared death, does not in some way accord with that of the bodhisattva:

> If the good Lord grants my desires, my heaven will be here on the earth until the end of the world. Yea, I would spend my heaven doing good on the earth. . . . When the angel will say, "Time is no more!" then will I rest, then will I rejoice, because the number of the elect will be whole and all will have entered into joy and into rest.[82]

By "heaven," we should here understand both a duration of time and the various graces that the Saint receives for distribution to others. This passage implies that in order to remain present to the world, she will

---

80. Orhan Pamuk, *The Black Book*, trans. Maureen Freely (New York: Vintage, 2006), 276.

81. The same is true in Ismailism, where the term is reserved for the Imam who substitutes his own spiritual authority for religious law. See Naṣīr al-Dīn al-Ṭūsī, *Paradise of Submission: A Medieval Treatise on Ismaili Thought*, trans. S. J. Badakhchani (New York: Tauris, 2005) §370, 418. Note that the resurrection of the dead is more precisely sketched out by baʿth. Sijistāni, for example, who deploys two separate notions, reserves qiyāmat for the Mahdi. Cf. Alī ibn ʿUthmān al-Jullābī al-Hujwīrī, *Kashf al-maḥjūb* (Leiden: Brill, 1911).

82. *Le carnet jaune* [The yellow notebook], July 17, 1897; cf. the letter of July 14, 1897, to Father Adolphe Roulland.

deprive herself of heavenly joys until she feels her task is complete. But as it is *her* heaven of which she would make such charitable use, this privation does not induce the tortures the bodhisattva declares himself ready to submit to. Thérèse's model is the resurrected Christ, the intercessor (see Hebrews 7:25), declaring, "And, lo, I am with you always, *even* unto the end of the world" (Matthew 28:20, emphasis added). But unlike Christ and the bodhisattva, Thérèse is not entirely in control of the fulfillment of her vow, which must first be approved by God, who alone possesses the supernatural means to put it to work. In addition, she must wait to know his answer, whereas the Three Nephites have theirs in the moment they make their request.

The vow, existentielly decisive, aims first of all to stimulate virtue and affirm will. Gandhi is explicit on this point: "A vow is an unwavering decision and helps us to defend ourselves against temptations. . . . All of humanity has learned, by experience, that without an unshakeable decision, progress is not possible."[83] This is why the treatise of Śāntideva is enriched by words of counsel addressed to the potential bodhisattva (concerning the means for either destroying the passions or achieving awakening on behalf of others),[84] even though it seems to have already framed the vow as if fidelity to it allowed the candidate to accumulate merit and, further, was ready to ensure its effective translation.

Hence the verse "From the moment the spirit embraces the tenacious idea of delivering the limitless mass of beings, though that spirit be sleepy or dissipated, the waves of its merits grow without ceasing, even as infinite as space."[85] Notwithstanding this attractive optimism,

---

83. Mahatma Gandhi, *Lettres à l'ashram* [Letters to the ashram], French trans. J. Herbert (Paris: Albin Michel, 1971), 100.

84. "Whether directly or indirectly, I should not do anything that is not for the benefit of others. And solely for the sake of sentient beings I should dedicate everything toward awakening." Śāntideva, *Bodhicaryāvatāra* V.101. "[I have] generated the awakening mind through wishing all beings to be happy" (ibid., VI.80).

85. Ibid., I.18–19 (translated from Finot's French as quoted by Hatem). It is important to note that in the Ten Stages (Daśabhūmika) Sutra (chapter 26 of *Flower Ornament Scripture*), the station of the vows is located in the first of ten lands, that of the supreme joy.

the spirit is still vulnerable to danger because of the dedication of self, and if it were to let itself be corrupted, this might place the universal good in peril: "Any failure of the Bodhisattva is very grave, for when he sins, it is the well-being of all others that he destroys."[86] Hence the necessity of vigilantly safeguarding his consciousness of the vow: "That which I have promised, I must bring about scrupulously; for if from today I do not work to that end, I will descend to lower and lower states."[87] The vow as existential decision comprises an engagement (a nonnegotiable token or security), an obligation to which one contracts oneself from the moment of a total deployment of conscience or consciousness, and a gift of self.

This gift, far from being made all at once, requires duration, not only because the subject himself is inscribed in time and is familiar with its phantasmagorias, but also because the vow is meant to benefit those who live inside history (not the eternal, in other words the everlasting, and not in some supratemporal reality, one outside of time).[88] Since it is constant, the nature of the vow itself requires an infinite duration of time.

Until every person can become a bodhisattva—taking up the vow as a sort of rallying cry, a call to transfiguration—the Mahdi and the Christ will not be reproduced, nor really even imitated (except wishfully or wistfully, as a sigh of envy). All three may be called vicars of humanity, but the Mahdi only in the sense of *being-beneath*.[89] The bodhisattva and the Christ alike substitute themselves for all of humanity in the sense of *being-in-the-place-of*—and for the same reason, although hardly by the same anthropological modality. Whereas the Eternal Word, becoming flesh, assumes human nature as such and in this way becomes the "New Adam," leader of the multitudes, the bodhisattva suffers only the

86. Ibid., IV.8 (translated from Finot's French as quoted by Hatem).

87. Ibid., IV.12 (translated from Finot's French as quoted by Hatem).

88. The bodies of the benevolent ones who constitute the Eight Immortals of the Taoist tradition, healing and helping all peoples, have not become eternal as a result of their generosity. One among them, Zhāng Guǒ Lǎo, in fact fell into his marvelous condition merely by chance when he accidentally drank an alchemist's broth.

89. The Mahdi helps those faithful to him and endeavors now and then to spare them their sufferings, but he does not take them upon himself. See Ibn Bābūya, *Kamāl al-dīn wa-tamām al-niʿmah*, 198.

liquefaction of ipseity and a displacement of the limits of virtue. Put another way, in Christianity human fulness models itself after the divine fulness of the second hypostasis of the Trinity; in Mahāyāna Buddhism, hypostasis must first dissolve itself so that the "I" can become all others. But precisely because of this emptiness, this last gesture is in everyone's reach, while because of the divine (and indissoluble) fulness of the Second Hypostasis, the Christian act is unique.[90] The Three Nephites naturally dwell below these figures because neither their ontological constitution nor their vocation authorizes them to attend to humanity except nominally, for their Messiah is already doing it effectively.

The reader will have noticed that in the cases analyzed here, the vow never tackles the question of the impossibility of its fulfillment. In Great Vehicle Buddhism, it is the order of the cosmos itself that is the deciding factor. In theistic religions, it is up to God to give his assent to the vow-as-request. The messianic existential becomes a supernatural existential the moment that natural kindness gains this greater value and sees itself from this moment on as having effect within the movements of Providence, the divine call duly ordaining it as of the kingdom.[91] A revelation given to Joseph Smith about the Saints pronounces accordingly, "They were set to be a light unto the world, and to be the saviors of men" (D&C 103:9).

---

90. Translator's footnote: In Trinitarian Christianity, each person of the Trinity is a "hypostasis" of the Trinity—a manifestation of its underlying reality. The Second Hypostasis of the Trinity is the Son.

91. For theists, the bodhisattva's attitude might be perceived as tarnished by pride, if pride consists of finding one's strength only in oneself. In return, the potential accusation that he reifies himself would not hold because he does not stop to recover himself but uses his merits to do new deeds.

2

Nistar

In the centuries that followed Christ's appearance to the Lehite remnant, wars multiplied, the revolt against God grew, and faith diminished such that "the Lord did take away his beloved disciples," the three Nephite disciples whose lives he had prolonged (Mormon 1:13; cf. Mormon 1:16). It is important to understand that he withdrew them from the bosom of the people who knew them, for they "did tarry in the land until the wickedness of the people was so great that the Lord would not suffer them to remain with the people; and whether they be upon the face of the land no man knoweth" (Mormon 8:10). Did the Lord take them to heaven, as he had done once before (see 3 Nephi 28:13–17)? This would seem to be suggested by the text, but I am inclined to believe that he was content to veil them from the eyes of the flesh. Yet even if they were removed, they would be brought back to earth, as the Book of Mormon also attests (see 3 Nephi 28:27–29).

The clandestineness of these Nephite pilgrims on the earth does not keep them from their ministry, nor does it prevent some of the faithful from meeting them.[1] Both Mormon and Moroni report seeing them and receiving instruction from them (see 3 Nephi 28:26; Mormon 8:11).

---

1. This is in contrast with Enoch and his brethren, of whom it is said in a revelation given to Joseph Smith that they are a city held in reserve until the day of righteousness (see D&C 45:11–12). Joseph Smith declared that Paul knew Enoch and was taught by him, but this phenomenon implies an extraordinary event (of a strictly horizontal dimension), be it the rapture of Paul or the condescension of Enoch. See Andrew F. Ehat and Lyndon W. Cook, eds., *The Words of Joseph Smith: The Contemporary Accounts*

Nevertheless, they remain hidden because they remain anonymous. Mormon, who would have lived in the fourth century, declares, "Behold, I was about to write the names of those who were never to taste of death, but the Lord forbade; therefore I write them not, for they are hid from the world" (3 Nephi 28:25). Their names will not echo through the ages, but their works will.[2] The name of the Mahdi is also to remain unspoken, such that anyone who utters it is considered miscreant;[3] his name is divulged only later.[4]

The Hasidic masters thought to divide the servants of righteousness in two classes: those who live discreetly among the *Hasidim*, and those known of the world. The condition of the *tzaddiq nistar* (one of the *Lamed-Vav Tzaddiqim*) would seem superior to these since, lost within the masses, he escapes the temptation to vanity. In this way, he resembles the *malāmatī* of Sufism, but is more moderate in that he does not attract reprobation in order to disguise his holiness. Some think it possible that the *nistar* is hidden even from himself so that, since he would not be the object of special distinction, he could fulfill his mission without giving it the least attention and without evincing exceptional heroism—especially if that mission consisted solely of existing in truth, in the simplest things, and not in a series of dazzling acts that would assure him wealth or consideration.[5] His essential nature is thus hidden, even from him, in a place so inscrutable as to be invisible, entirely covered over by an accessory nature: not of the thaumaturge or

---

of the Nauvoo Discourses of the Prophet Joseph (Provo, UT: Religious Studies Center, Brigham Young University, 1980), 41.

2. More precisely, the names of the three are in this list: Nephi, Jonas son of Nephi, Timothy, Mathoni, Mathonihah, Kumen, Kumenonhi, Jeremiah, Shemnon, Jonas, Zedekiah, and Isaiah (see 3 Nephi 19:4).

3. See Ibn Bābūya, *Kamāl al-dīn wa-tamām al-niʿmah* (Beirut: Al-Aʿlamī, 2004), 587–88. Cf. Muhammad ibn Ibrahim al-Nuʿmānī, *Kitāb al-ghaybat* (Qom: n. p., 2005), 300.

4. The Mahdi bears the name of the Prophet of Islam; cf. al-Nuʿmānī, *Kitāb al-ghaybat*, 94, 187.

5. This would happen only *in extremis*, as in the Hasidic story of Rabbi Raphael of Belz, who discovers that the nondescript Isaac Leib, whom he thought a sinner, is in reality a perfect man, to whom the elements themselves submit.

nonconformist, nor of the dregs of the earth, but of a perfect normality over which the gaze of the other would skitter and slide. His is a righteousness careless of renown, a virtue mingled with common humanity.

The concealment of the Mahdi, by contrast, is peculiar and does not tarnish his purpose.[6] In the first place, he takes pains to hide himself in order to deprive his enemies of any handhold. It is said that he sinks underground, communicating with the faithful from there, for a time, through the mediation of four representatives.[7] It is also said that his body remains unseen (*lā yurā jismuhū*), whereas he himself can observe others,[8] suggesting either a supernatural veiling or a transmutation as needed, both of which are evoked at will in crediting stories of encounters with him who, hidden, would reside in a parallel (if not a superior) world of the most subtle quality.

But the latter is only a hypothesis conveyed by the Shaykhi School, and is largely dismissed by the more accepted suggestion that he is in fact visible but unknown, living alongside us without us suspecting him.

---

6. The following sentence is ascribed to the First Imam: "The earth is never left without a defense, either known by all or hidden to all." Ibn Bābūya, *Kamāl al-dīn wa-tamām al-niʿmah*, 276 (translated from Hatem's French rendering).

7. This underground space is much like the cavern where the Seven Sleepers were immured (become for them the image of a protective hollow), so much so that the Mahdi remains conscious of time and does not intend, when the moment comes, to return to its windowless and ahistorical walls in order to place his soul there (as the Sleepers do in the *Mīmar* of Jacob of Sarug on the Children of Ephesus, though they are, thanks to the mercy of a resurrecting God, merely sleeping). See also Gregory of Tours, *Glory of the Martyrs* XCV. It is noteworthy that in order to justify the Mahdi's longevity, Shiʿite writers put forward the legend, echoed in the Qurʾan, of the Sleepers who can pass through a kind of hibernation; cf. Abū Jaʿfar al-Tūsī, *Kitāb al-ghaybat* (Beirut: Muassasat dār al-kitāb, 1988), 73. They know neither the dormition of Abimelech, which lasted seventy years (see 4 Baruch 5:30), nor, of course, the sleep of Endymion, which will last as long as the earth and sky. In his commentary on verse 9 of "The Cavern" surah, the Tafsīr of Qāshānī makes of the children walled up alive the seven perfect ones who balance the cosmos.

8. Cf. Muhammad Yaʿqūb al-Kulaynī, *Usūl al-kāfī* (Beirut: Dāt al-adwā, 1992),1:394, 400.

He moves from city to city in order to avoid discovery,[9] goes to Mecca during the pilgrimage, and helps his followers when they are in difficulty.[10] This tangible presence, according to Muḥammad Bāqir al-Ṣadr, gives the Twelfth Imam advantage over all other claimants.[11] However, something in him is not concealed, something that is pointedly protected by his inglorious self-concealment: his unyielding opposition to established power, from which he has always freed himself. The Imams who came before him owed allegiance, in effect, to usurping caliphs, something he would not intentionally allow himself by virtue of the rebellion he will one day have to lead. While he waits for that day, his portion is a splendid isolation, whether one attributes wives and progeny to him or not. Some describe him as erratic, solitary, hunted.[12] Does he not risk being denied or forgotten as a result of the shadow of an earth that, Lamartine would say, is cast on its star?[13]

It is as if the two phases of the Three Nephites' career were distributed in the two hypotheses of the Imamites. The theory of the Mahdi's sojourn in the imaginal world—the green isle, Qāf mountain, or better, the Land of Nowhere (*Na-kōjā-abād*) in which time is of a psychic or subtle nature (*latīf*)—corresponds to the removal of the Three Nephites in the face of persecution. Their terrestrial life corresponds to the theory of the Mahdi's existence among men, though his deportment in our times is inscrutable (*kathīf*). We do know that the Three Nephites already benefit from a transformation that shields them from their enemies: cast three times into a furnace, they suffered no harm (3 Nephi 28:21). Their basic diet was also altered. But according to the second

---

9. Cf. Muḥammad Bāqir al-Ṣadr, *Tārīkh al-ghaybah al-sughrá* (Qom: n.p., 2006), 37.

10. Cf. Hussayn al-Tabarsī al-Nūrī, *Al-Najm al-thāqib fī ahwāl alimām al-hujjat al-ghā'ib* (n.p.: n.p., n.d.), 2:332.

11. Muḥammad Bāqir al-Ṣadr, *Bahth hawl al-Mahdī* (Qom: n.p., 1996), 55. I note the Shaykhist theory of the men of the invisible (*rijāl al-ghayb*): the Mahdi's friends (*awliyā'*) unknown to the public.

12. Muhammad ibn Jarīr al-Tabarī, *Dalā'il al-Imāmat* (Beirut: Al-a'lamī, 1988), 285.

13. Cf. verse 105 of Lamartine's "Hymne au Christ."

theory, that of being hidden in plain sight, such is not the case for the Mahdi, who, his longevity set aside, is submitted, like the thirty-six righteous men, to the same empirical and spatiotemporal conditions as men made of common clay. It is not clear, for example, that the Three Nephites endure hunger and thirst. Given that their suffering is only moral or spiritual and can only be understood as a simple result of their solicitude for men, it has no redemptive reach, unlike that of the Christ.[14]

Precisely because of his vulnerability to the conditions of mortality, the Mahdi has protected himself by occultation since his early childhood. And those through whom he speaks apparently resent attempts to injure him because they have him pray that those who weave traps for him will fall into their own nets.[15] Justice trumps charity from the moment one promises to punish with absolute severity those who walk in error and crime: a consequence of a policy of predilection that wields condemnation. In Buddhism, it is the bodhisattva who weaves nets to catch the beasts[16] and reprobates he intends to save: "He enters all the hells of all the universes he visits to succor the damned until he can free them."[17] Śāntideva exclaims, "It is essential to do good, even to our worst enemies."[18] Indeed, among the exceptional beings who are the object of this study, only the bodhisattva, in his great grace, cherishes and

14. Concerning Christ's expiatory sacrifice, Mormon doctrine largely conforms to Christian orthodoxy (though with a particular emphasis on Gethsemane). See by way of example 2 Nephi 2:7–9; Mosiah 3:11; 3 Nephi 11:14; Articles of Faith 1:3.

15. Muḥammad ibn al-Ḥasan Mahdī, *Adʿiyat al-Imām al-Mahdī* (Beirut: Dār al-Murtadā, 2000), 61. The sources often insist that the Mahdi will use violence when he reveals himself; cf. al-Nuʿmānī, *Kitāb al-ghaybat*, 159. Mercy will not be his strength (ibid., 237). It is said that Allah declares that he will avenge himself through the Mahdi for the massacre at Karbalah (ibid., 96).

16. "May all animals be free from the fear of being eaten by one another." Śāntideva, *Bodhicaryāvatāra* X.16.

17. See *The Holy Teaching of Vimalakīrti: A Mahāyāna Scripture*, trans. Robert A. F. Thurman (University Park: Pennsylvania State University Press, 1976), 70 (translated from Carré's French as quoted by Hatem); Śāntideva, *Bodhicaryāvatāra*, X.15 (translated from Finot's French as quoted by Hatem).

18. Śāntideva, *Bodhicaryāvatāra*, VI.120 (translated from Finot's French as quoted by Hatem).

seeks out suffering,[19] whereas the righteous men take it upon themselves without knowing the suffering of the world.[20] Far from being immune to pain, the bodhisattva enters into the play of absolute passivity, laying himself open, in an act of propitiation, and he delivers himself to all in an everlasting passion.

Fear, therefore, is not the reason that the bodhisattva might conceal himself. First of all, he does not fear death; he seeks out vexations. Second, he disguises himself only for the work of conversion, a little like the Christian God who comes incognito into the world but with an advantage. Unlike the Christian God, who is irreversibly tied to his human body, the bodhisattva acquires magical powers—among them the power to show himself as he chooses in any stage of life, as any sort of person, or in the form of gods or things.[21] Since he understands that all is spirit, he is able to master the elements, borrow various bodies, and move through walls so easily that it is said his work meets with no impediment.[22]

Is it not tempting to qualify comments about the bodhisattva's pain, given the miracles of which he is capable as a person who fulfills more than his strict duty to humankind? Has he not, in the manner of the Three Nephites, taken possession of a new body? Ought we not to have doubts about the simply metaphorical or purely moral nature of the sickness that Vimalakīrti professes, a sickness that prompts the Buddha to send eight thousand Bodhisattvas, five hundred Auditors, and one hundred thousand men and gods to enquire after his health? This is the explanation he gives:

> My sickness comes from ignorance and the thirst for existence and it will last as long as do the sicknesses of all living beings. Were all living beings to be free from sickness, I also would not be sick. Why? For the bodhisattva, the world consists only of living

---

19. "I should indeed be solely joyful toward such suffering that dispels the harms of all." Śāntideva, *Bodhicaryāvatāra* VI.75.

20. Cf. André Schwarz-Bart, *The Last of the Just*, trans. Stephen Becker (New York: Atheneum, 1961), 52–61.

21. *Holy Teaching of Vimalakīrti*, 69–72.

22. *The Laṅkāvatāra Sūtra* 2.26; *The Flower Ornament Scripture* III.5.

> beings, and sickness is inherent in living in the world. Were all living beings free of sickness, the bodhisattva also would be free of sickness.[23]

It is clear that the bodhisattva Vimalakīrti's sickness springs from two sources: existence and vicarious substitution. But does this necessarily mean that he offers up his body to wrongdoing only in a metaphorical sense? After all, moral suffering rarely fails to present physically. Indeed, it is said that as soon as the bodhisattva Avalokiteshvara saw the immense misery of creatures, his head exploded from the pain. From the scattered fragments, nine new heads were fashioned for him by the Buddha Amitābha.

The eschatological tension resides in *homo absconditus*'s way of being, in his capacity as vestige of the Unconditioned among us (the *Bikerbenu Yahweh* of the Jewish tradition). If he had been continually manifest, a theology of presence would have prevailed over a theology of hope (which occurs when churches are built or the Imam sits in judgment and governance, as among the Isma'ilis). In order to be the inviolable figure of hope at the heart of history, the Imam puts in crisis all political theology adapted to the world. This is what Twelver Shiʿism realizes[24] and thus refutes the Fatimid Caliphate not only on the basis of a false lineage but equally for the simple observation that it in no way established the reign of justice. Hence the axiom that, added to eschatological uncertainty, leads to quietism: "Every standard raised before that of Qa'im belongs to a tyrant."[25] And if the Mahdi seemed cast back to the periphery of history, it could only be as its principal actor, not as its privileged witness. If he is not its center, it is because of

---

23. *Holy Teaching of Vimalakīrti*, 43.

24. Cf. Jad Hatem, *Eléments de théologie politique* [Elements of political theology] (Paris: L'Harmattan, 2005), especially chapters 1 and 5.

25. Al-Nuʿmānī, *Kitāb al-ghaybat*, 115. Shaykhist Imamism teaches that it is forbidden to launch a holy war during the Occultation (cf. Muhammad Karim Khan, *Al-Risālat aljihādiyya*). The danger of (alcoholic) drink is that which Philothée O'Neddy (Théophile Dondey de Santeny) calls "*le philtre endormeur de l'espoir*," or "the potion which lulls hope to sleep" (from "*Nécropolis*," 14).

the ahistorical character of the situation, seeing that he is alone in both initiating the decisive instant and introducing the novelty. It is the entire history of salvation that is on hold, a history so little coordinated with world history since the Occultation that the first act of the Mahdi will be to abolish world history, not to fulfill it.

I have indicated that although the Sunnis recognize a Mahdi, they do not identify him with the Twelfth Imam (in whose existence they do not believe), but rather with the Son of Mary, who will—as the end of time approaches[26]—return as impartial judge and vanquish the enemies of true religion. They explain his exemption from death by referring to the Qurʾan, which does not admit his crucifixion. However, his career does not continue among human communities because the Book specifies that Allah raised him unto himself (see 4:158). When the Son of Mary comes, he will descend from where he resides: the second heaven (or the fourth, according to other sources). It is the use of the word *nuzūl* (descent) that indicates, according to commentators, that Jesus lives in the supraterrestrial region.[27] Indeed, if he had lived on the earth, one commentator points out, he would have been obliged to find Muhammad and support his cause.[28] Ibn ʿArabī assigns him a particular destiny in attributing to him the eminent title "Seal of Universal Holiness." He conceives the existence of four pillars bodily present in the world until the day of the resurrection: Idris, Jesus, Elijah, and Khodr. By them, Allah preserves faith, holiness, prophecy, and mission.[29] In reality, Idris and Jesus reside in celestial spheres, but these are considered by Ibn ʿArabī as part of the cosmos. The Judeo-Christian tradition holds that Elijah and Enoch (the Idris of Islam) have also been raised up.

---

26. There are Sunni texts that have Muhammad saying he was waiting for this imminent descent; cf. Hindī, *Muntakhab* (Cairo: n.p., 1895), 6:55–56.

27. For an example taken from the Shiʿite tradition: Imam al-Baqir would have said that the Son of Mary "will descend to the world (*ilâ al-dunyâ*) on the day of Resurrection." Muhammad Baqir al-Majlesi, *Bihār al-anwār* (Beirut: al-Wafāʾ, 1983), 14:530.

28. Cf. Al-Hāfiz Abū al-Fadl al-Hasanī, *ʿAqīdat ahl al-Islām fī nuzūl ʿĪsā ʿalayhi al-salām* (Beirut: ʿAlam al-kutub, 1986), 30.

29. Ibn ʿArabi, *The Meccan Revelations*, 2 vols., trans. William C. Chittick, James Winston Morris, Cyrille Chodkiewicz, and Denis Gril (New York: Pir, 2002–2004).

Elijah must return as a precursor of the Messiah, per Malachi 3:22–23 (see Matthew 17:10–12). The Message of La Salette[30] announces that Enoch and Elijah, "filled with the Holy Spirit, will preach with the force of God."[31] Mormon doctrine also has it that Elijah was preserved from death for several centuries until he had accomplished all the missions that had been entrusted to him (see D&C 110:13).[32] Enoch's case is even more spectacular, since not only was he raised up to God, but, according to Mormon belief, he was raised up together with the entire city he had built, with all its inhabitants (see Moses 7:69).

In conclusion, the Son of Mary is tangential to the paradigm of human messianicity: although he no longer moves among people, he plays a role in the conservation of the human world and remains present to it, ready to appear once more. Though it does not confer upon Jesus the position of Mahdi, one may remember that the Shiʿite doctrine allows for his return as an auxiliary of the Twelfth Imam: a meeting of the two hidden from men—one among them, the other in a heaven or in a sphere of the imaginal world; a means to proceed to a convergence and not merely a harnessing of legacy. Does the Mahdi not sometimes resemble Jesus physically as well as morally? Is it not said that he comes again (*lahu rajʿat*) after the manner of the Son of Mary?[33]

Katarina Frostenson pronounces: "We fell the forest and the bare isle makes its way in the light. All our disquiet yields before the form that appears."[34]

---

30. Translator's note: Hatem has reference here to an apparition of Mary in La Salette, France, in 1846.

31. Cf. Léon Bloy, *Celle qui pleure, Appendice l'apparition et le secret* [She who cries: Appendix to the apparition and the secret] (Paris: Société du Mercure de France, 1908), especially chapter 3.

32. Doctrine and Covenants 110:14 recalls the prophecy of Malachi; see also 3 Nephi 24–25.

33. Al-Majlesi, *Bihār al-anwār*, 52:226.

34. Katarina Frostenson, *Canal*, trans. Christofer Bjurström (Beuvry: Maison de la poésie d'Amay, 1998), 131 (translated from the French).

3

Kerygma

THE THREE NEPHITES DISTINGUISH THEMSELVES from the thirty-six righteous men and the Imam by their proselytism:[1]

> And behold they will be among the Gentiles, and the Gentiles shall know them not. They will also be among the Jews, and the Jews shall know them not. And it shall come to pass, when the Lord seeth fit in his wisdom that they shall minister unto all the scattered tribes of Israel, and unto all nations, kindreds, tongues and people, and shall bring out of them unto Jesus many souls, that their desire may be fulfilled, and also because of the convincing power of God which is in them. And they are as the angels of God, and if they shall pray unto the Father in the name of Jesus they can show themselves unto whatsoever man it seemeth them good. Therefore, great and marvelous works shall be wrought by them, before the great and coming day when all people must surely stand before the judgment-seat of Christ; Yea even among the Gentiles shall there be a great and marvelous work wrought by them, before that judgment day. (3 Nephi 28:27–32)

The Book of Mormon does not establish a causal connection between anonymity and the work of conversion. That is, the method of conversion

1. Conversion to God is key to the mission given to Joseph Smith, to whom Christ says, "And if it so be that you should labor all your days in crying repentance unto this people, and bring, save it be one soul unto me, how great shall be your joy with him in the kingdom of my Father!" (D&C 18:15).

does not seem to rest on remaining hidden, a condition that would profit nothing but safety.

This connection, however, is explicit in the case of the bodhisattva, who is not content merely to succor people and to be responsible for them,[2] but takes great pains to lead them to safety:

> They intentionally become courtesans in order to win men over, and, having caught them with the hook of desire, they establish them in the Buddha-gnosis. . . . They fearlessly behold those who are masters to be served, and they become their servants or slaves. . . . They demonstrate all activities, whichever possibly may be a means to make beings delight in the Dharma. . . . Having perfected an infinite wisdom, they liberate an infinitude of living beings.[3]

In passing into a region of shadow and illusion, the Mahdi has no plans to convert others. We have seen that, according to one tradition, his disappearance made the danger of apostasy weigh heavily on those Shiʿites gnawed by impatience and doubt. Would it sift them? Could it be the means of discovering who is a *substantially* authentic believer? These questions are answered in the doctrine professed by the Fifth Imam, who desired that the Imams and the hearts of their followers be made of the more noble part of the firmament so that they might yearn naturally after their Imam in contrast with their enemies, whose hearts are drawn to an infernal substance.[4] In superimposing these two givens, the test becomes a factor in setting aside all those who will not truly partake of the celestial substance. Inversely, potential Shiʿites turn freely toward their Imam. In any event, the teaching attributed to Imam Muhammad al-Bāqir cannot nourish the hope of a voluntary and universal rallying to the sacred cause.

---

2. "The love that is effort because it takes responsibility for all living beings." *The Holy Teaching of Vimalakīrti: A Mahāyāna Scripture*, trans. Robert A. F. Thurman (University Park: Pennsylvania State University Press, 1976), 57.

3. Ibid., 71–72. It is equally noteworthy that the bodhisattva goes to gaming houses to save gamblers and to houses of pleasure to reveal the dangers of carnal desire (ibid., 21).

4. In Muhammad Yaʿqūb al-Kulaynī, *Usūl al-kāfī* (Beirut: Dāt al-adwā, 1992), 2:7.

And yet, is there not room to think that he who sustains the world merely by his holy presence (who gives himself, therefore, to the ontological good, that which makes God prefer being to nothingness and privilege mercy over anger)[5] would necessarily develop a heart totally and unconditionally receptive? The degree of the self-effacement of the *nistar* would be in the measure of this receptivity. One may believe Katarina Frostenson: "Of myself I am nothing, but in the desert I am that which may contain all.[6]

5. These two traits are equivalent for F. W. J. Schelling: it is in subordinating anger to love that the Eternal changes the force of contraction into the foundation of a force of expansion.

6. Katarina Frostenson, *Canal*, trans. Christofer Bjurström (Beuvry: Maison de la poésie d'Amay, 1998), 123 (translated from the French).

4

Contemporaneity

IF THE EMPHASIS ON THE POSTPONEMENT of heavenly glory can be shifted from the actual supplicant to whoever imagines or thinks it (from the Three Nephites to Joseph Smith, for example), a new concept intervenes in the link with the original apostolate: that of contemporaneity. Not being a contemporary of the incarnate God, like the beloved disciple (immediate contemporaneity), and instead of turning back to a tradition that transmits the possibility of salvation (mediate contemporaneity), Smith conceives a redoubled immediate contemporaneity that makes him the immediate contemporary of those (the apostles) who were the immediate contemporaries of Christ moving among men. Even if he had not mentioned a meeting with John and even though he did not mention a meeting with the Three Nephites, the possibility of such a meeting could not be set aside—and it remains a possibility for everyone, even today, and a way to be in better communication with the event than across an uncertain transmission.[1] Similarly, neither Mormon nor Moroni was present during the appearance of the resurrected Christ to the Nephites.

I hazard the hypothesis that the reason for which an encounter with the Three Nephites holds no place in Smith's apostolic plan[2] is that he

1. Advocates of this immediate contemporaneity, redoubled or not, may put to suspicion the apostolic (and pontifical) and Fatimid successions, as well as that of the first Eleven legatees in Twelver Shiʿism.

2. An allusion in an article of April 1842 takes a satirical turn. Referring to certain luminaries of the church, Smith mentions the case of a member who declared he must

achieved still another contemporaneity, irreducible to any of the three just mentioned—all of which might be located along the line of temporal horizontality. It was not enough for Smith to be the translator of the Book of Mormon, however original a figure that made him. He rises to the stature of prophet by receiving revelations directly, becoming the direct contemporary of Christ vertically. The result is a rupture in the line of temporal horizontality (a rupture not present in the discovery of the Book of Mormon, seeing that it was merely buried in the earth). In effect, it is the supratemporal that comes to meet Smith in the person of the Father and the Son or angels. He establishes contact with the beyond practically at will, as can be seen in his autobiography.

The paradigm of the longevity of Christ's direct contemporary in horizontality (John or the Three Nephites) weakens from the moment the direct contemporary establishes himself in verticality. After the death of their founder, the Latter-day Saints had the opportunity to strengthen the paradigm of horizontal longevity by conceiving, for example, a system similar to that which the Mahdi put in place during the Minor Occultation: communicating with the faithful via the intermediary of a deputy, a system that would have allowed the Three Nephites to oversee the direction of the community. But the Latter-day Saints preferred to follow Smith's second inspiration in safeguarding the gift of prophecy from one president of the church to the next, such that direct contemporaneity in verticality is maintained until Christ's return. With the establishment of the church, institutional logic won out over sporadic and anarchic shifts. In consequence, the paradigm of the Three Nephites does not seem to have traction in Mormon doctrine. As with the Eight Immortals of Taoism and the Mahdi,[3] folklore has taken

---

be conducted to the Rocky Mountains by the Three Nephites, but they did not keep the appointment. Joseph Smith, "Try the Spirits," *Times and Seasons* 3 (April 1, 1842): 743–47. Michael Hicks urges caution in assigning editorial authorship during this period, as Smith often worked in collaboration with others. See "Joseph Smith, W. W. Phelps, and the Poetic Paraphrase of 'The Vision,'" *Journal of Mormon History* 20 (Fall 1994): 68.

3. There are several accounts of very surprising encounters with the Mahdi in Muhammad Bāqir al-Majlesi, *Bihār al-anwār* (Beirut: al-Wafā', 1983), 52:159–80.

hold[4] of the accounts of people who have seen them, been taught by them, or even been succored or healed under their care.[5] It must have seemed strange to his followers that the Prophet Joseph Smith did not contribute, by personal testimony, to the saga of the Three Nephites. This is why such a testimony was attributed to him later on.[6]

In the *Midrash on Lamentations*, it is said that the Messiah was born at the same moment as the destruction of the temple,[7] which is not to say that he had already manifested himself as the Messiah. The theory of his longevity would not easily be discarded, in support of

---

4. The same is true of Mormon literature. In Orson Scott Card's novel *Speaker for the Dead*, the protagonist Ender, who bears the burden of human guilt, is still young after three thousand years, thanks to his interstellar voyages. See Card, *Speaker for the Dead* (New York: Tor, 1994).

5. On these microhistories, see Hector Lee, *The Three Nephites: The Substance and Significance of the Legend in Folklore* (Albuquerque: University of New Mexico Press, 1949); and Douglas Beardall and Jewel Beardall, *About the Three Nephites* (Provo, UT: LDS Books Publications, 1992). As a case in point, it is attested that the Three appear suddenly in a room, without passing through the door, in order to care for a gravely ill child. The phraseology that they appear "out of nowhere" and disappear in like manner becomes something of a refrain. To my mind, the touching story of a woman whose husband had been sent on a mission to Germany deserves special mention. On a winter morning, an old man knocks at her door and tells her he is hungry. Even though she is impoverished, she gives him a loaf of bread wrapped in some colorful fabric. The man goes away without leaving a single track in the snow. When her husband returns several years later, she discovers the same bit of fabric in his suitcase. One Christmas evening, when he was penniless, a stranger offered him some bread (Beardall and Beardall, *About the Three Nephites*, 125–26). There are comparable accounts about the Mahdi, whose fortuitous appearances meet the needs of the poor and the lost.

6. Cf. Bruce Dana, *The Three Nephites and Other Translated Beings* (Springville, UT: Cedar Fort, 2003), 51–53. The author, though Mormon, invites both circumspection and doubt. Brigham Young, Joseph Smith's successor as the head of the church, announced in 1859 that some strangers would visit the members in order to shed light on the mysteries of the faith. He said the souls of the saints would tremble on that occasion like those of the disciples on the road to Emmaus. See *Journal of Discourses*, 26 vols. (London: Latter-day Saints' Book Depot, 1854–1886), 6:194–95. Even though the Three Nephites are not explicitly mentioned, one can assume that Young spoke about them.

7. *Lamentations Rabbah* 1:51.

which one invokes the longevity of the first humans, "for life is God's."[8] According to another tradition, he has already appeared in the soul of Adam, suggesting that he is reincarnated in every age: in David, in Moses, and so on.[9] These traditions offer assurance that the seed of salvation is always already planted or germinates as a kind of instantiated replica at the dismantling of the sacrificial cult such that another modality of the divine presence is ensured. This does not make of the Jew the contemporary of a promise but of its fulfillment; the Jew awaits the Messiah's appearance to the plain view and knowledge of the world. This is a new way to conceive the *already-there-and-not-yet*, but it helps us comprehend a way of crossing history. The legend that the Messiah was born on the day of the temple's destruction persists: scarcely born, the winds carried him far from his mother's breast, and he wanders unknown from nation to nation, redemption occurring only once he has been to all of them.[10]

The case of the Imam-Messiah of Druzism completes the tableau.[11] The Druze teach that in order to escape persecutions, the Imam-Messiah withdrew from the world nearly one thousand years ago to a region called the Oases, the location of which is unknown, and from which he will not return except to establish his rule. The uniqueness of the Imam-Messiah's case consists of the fact that to sustain the idea of constant presence—by turns hidden and manifest—Druzism need not imagine, as Shiʿism must, a succession of prophets and Imams because it accepts the theory of metempsychosis.

---

8. Ramban (Nachmanides), *Writings and Discourses*, 2 vols., trans. Charles B. Chavel (New York: Shilo, 1978), 2:668 (32).

9. Cf. Gershom G. Scholem, *Major Trends in Jewish Mysticism* (New York: Schocken, 1961), 278. On the reincarnations of the Messiah, son of Joseph, in the Lurianic Kabbalah, see Hayyim Vital, *Traité de la Révolution des âmes* [Treatise on the revolution of souls] (Milan, Archè, 1987), 288, 402; and Moshe Idel, *Messianic Mystics* (New Haven: Yale University Press, 1998), 167.

10. For Franz Rosenzweig, this means the veiling of the Jewish Messiah in Christianity as revelation spread among the pagans. See Rosenzweig's *Foi et savoir* [Faith and knowledge] (Paris: Vrin, 2001), 77.

11. Cf. Jad Hatem, *Dieu en guise d'homme dans le druzisme* [God in the guise of man in Druzism] (Paris: Librarie de l'Orient, 2006).

The most striking fact is that he who messianically endures for so long anchors the actual always and for all in the evental. He does not seek to mock destiny, and seeks even less to bandy with time. Of course, the bodhisattva's time passes to allow the linearity of *saṃsāra*, the wheel of reincarnation. The same does not apply to messianic time, which is haunted, even besieged, by *kairos*, the opportune moment, engorged by fulness and perfectly significant: qualitative, existentiell, multifaceted time, susceptible to interruption in every instant in order to understand the curve of a decisive turning. This distended time does not get stuck in its own course as long as the incognito is shielded from those who have inserted themselves, not as challengers, but as fulfillers. But such a moment never adequately fulfills the hope and expectation dependent upon a utopian promise to exorcise evil.

The contemporaneity of the Three Nephites cannot ignore eschatological expectation, for their duration unravels a time-for-others charged with guaranteeing the continuation of history. The future dwells in coming. What mediates between worlds is the creative synthesis of the promise and of time (itself a combination of spirit and of world) such that history has at its immanent center a purely human standard-bearer.

The Mahdi is just as much a mediator, being, the texts say, the taut cord between men and God.[12] However, his temporality necessitates some amendments. Even though he was not contemporary with the origins of Islam, he very nearly was. This is a serviceable argument. The Shiʿite theologian Muhammad Bāqir al-Ṣadr underlines, for example, the advantage that the Mahdi was born *near* the sources of Islam—before rising up against the values of a pernicious civilization, it was good, for fear of contamination, that his personality be formed entirely in other times.[13] Besides an accumulation of time, his is a mentality made more and more awkward by relation to the present: an intellectual noncurrency in good taste. But there is another consideration. It is

12. Cf. Muhammad ibn Ibrahim al-Nuʿmānī, *Kitāb al-ghaybat* (Qom: n. p., 2005), 37, 49.

13. Muḥammad Bāqir al-Ṣadr, *Bahth hawl al-Mahdī* (Qom: n.p., 1996), 88.

accepted among the Shiʿites that the Imams were born of a light created before the world.[14] Their germ, deposited in Adam, moves through generational lines until its gradual fruition in the Twelve, who are one in essence. What distinguishes the preexistence of the Imams from that of other men is primarily that their ontological worthiness is superior, and secondarily that they do not lose self-awareness in their incarnations.

The question of contemporaneity requires a change of inflection in the case of the bodhisattva. By virtue of their reincarnations, all creatures were always already his contemporaries. This was useful to Gendun Gyatso, the second Dalai Lama (alternatively known in Tibetan Buddhism as a partial incarnation of Avalokiteshavra), in founding universal compassion. One might recall Śāntideva's method appealing to the inversion of *me* and *others*. The Dalai Lama's trick consists of developing in his soul a feeling of universal recognition. Remember, he suggests, your mother and all her kindnesses and the innumerable sacrifices to which she consented. Was she not ready to do anything and all for you, even at the risk of public disgrace? From there he passes to relatives and friends. Have they not of necessity been your mothers in some other reincarnation? Must not one therefore return that love for the extreme benevolence they have shown? The argument is equally valid for the multitudes. Is it not right to be compassionate to them? What to say, then, of enemies? We must think of them as blinded by their rebirths. They do not realize that they were your mothers and you were theirs. It is right to act in their regard as with a mother who, suddenly taken by madness, assaults you.[15] The beauty of the idea must not conceal that it rests on a pre-Mahayanist psychology that sees that the ego is maintained even as Śāntideva undermines it.

It follows from omnitemporality that the bodhisattva is hostage to all others in that he can only be progressively delivered from time by their entrance into nirvana. His case is aggravated by the fact that he

---

14. Cf. Ibn Bābūya, *ʿIlal al-sharāʾiʿ wa-l-ahkām* (Najaf: n.p., 1966), 135–36.

15. Text reproduced in the anthology of S. Bercholz and S. Chodzin Kohn, *Pour comprendre le Bouddhisme* [Understanding Buddhism] (Paris: Laffont, 1993), chapter 14.

remembers in every detail all of his prior existences.[16] Without metempsychosis,[17] the Three Nephites and the Mahdi see their commitment passed on to the offspring of those for whom they are responsible and whom they survive.

16. *The Flower Ornament Scripture* III.5.

17. Joseph Smith formally rejected belief in metempsychosis, or the transmigration of souls, during an 1835 conversation with one "Robert Mathias." See Dean C. Jessee, Mark Ashurst-McGee, and Richard L. Jensen, eds., *Journals, Volume 1: 1832–1839*, vol. 1 of the Journals series of *The Joseph Smith Papers*, ed. Dean C. Jessee, Ronald K. Esplin, and Richard Lyman Bushman (Salt Lake City: Church Historian's Press, 2008), 95. Ultra-Shiʿism accepts it. Twelver Shiʿism recognizes metemphotosis, to borrow a clarifying term from Mohammad Ali Ami-Moezzi (*The Divine Guide in Early Shiʿism: The Sources of Esotericism in Islam*, trans. David Streight [Albany, NY: SUNY, 1994], 75–77), which is to say a transmission from one Imam to another of the primordial light, though the soul of one Imam is not the soul of another. There is certainly an archetypal Imam, but those who appear on the world stage, although they come from the same source, are not the same person.

5

Nephite-Mahdite Time

BECAUSE WE FALL SHORT OF BEING, we hurry toward the future, conceived as a dimension of fulfillment. It is not quite the same for the Three Nephites, the bodhisattva, and the Mahdi inasmuch as they would have already realized their essence had it not been for their concern for others. What is more, their temporality implies a differently accented transcendence: time in equilibrium, certainly, as it lengthens and weaves itself together with the time of men that goes its customary way, but unstable as it assures the link between the present and the Absolute (Advent or Nirvāna). If these figures anticipate something, it is not death, but the irruption of the kingdom or perfect peace. It is properly the time of a hidden, immanent presence (and not that of an interim, as is the case with the Christian tradition), but which is not merely an inflection of *being-with*. In effect, it is not sufficient to say that it is because they possess the constitution *to-be-with* that they set themselves apart or hide from the gazes of the malevolent as well as the faithful. To advance *being-toward* and *being-for*, they place themselves in a wrinkle in time with such intensity that the thread of finite life, woven into the details, is exceeded such that history allows just such a flawless human gaze—at once submerged and afloat in the flow of time—to conform history to its eternal designs regardless of the too-small souls,[1]

1. "Why wear your feeble soul with plans for eternity?," *Horace's Odes and Epodes*, trans. David Mulroy (Ann Arbor: University of Michigan Press, 1994), 111 (2.11).

all in following its tours and detours[2] (scansions of a like identity and occasional alternation in route and return).[3]

What I call Nephite-Mahdite time—constituted, at the heart of the difference between the actual and the possible, by the union in the *present* of being and of before-occurring [*devant-advenir*]—is the controlling thread that, linking the initial and the terminal, tempers what is dolorous, incomprehensible, or scandalous in the distension between them. Do not the Ismaili Imams do much the same? Certainly. But since they rearrange and occupy the front of the stage every time, for a given moment, they do not possess that body which, Sándor Márai would say, contains the enigma of time.[4] And since they can also suspend the law of their own leader and usher in the kind of messianic time that gives precedence to purely spiritual religion, they change the very tenor of expectation. Now the perception of the duration of time varies necessarily with the modifications made to expectation. There are, therefore, several ways to forge a unity in the present of the future and of the possible. Nephite-Mahdite time subordinates *being-for* to *being-beneath*, such that the hidden presence becomes—to the one enduring who considers the course of the world from two points of view, immanent and transcendent—the memory of the Unconditioned in the circumstances of world history.[5]

A secret doctrine and the science of the significance of Arabic letters (*jafr*) are passed from one Imam to another. But equally significant is that the inspired Book given through Fatima is supposed to contain a

2. Translator's note: I retain Hatem's "*tours et détours*" for its playfulness. The English *tour* is synonymous with *journey* here.

3. *Corso e ricorso*, in Vico's vocabulary. A return to barbarism and apostasy (essentially equivalent terms) is frequent, according to the Book of Mormon.

4. Sándor Márai, *Embers*, trans. Carol Brown Janeway (New York: Vintage, 2002), 9–15.

5. Even though he shares in equal measure the memory of the Unconditioned, the Wandering Jew, as a figure of despair, experiences it as a burden that obliges him to nothing and of which he dreams of ridding himself. The Jew Pär Lagerkvist imagines in *The Death of Ahasuerus* undoing the spell that binds him to earthly existence by discovering that he, like the Crucified, is the victim of an inexorable god. But he has not resolved the dilemma of knowing for what (or for whom) to live.

complete account of future events.[6] Yet this is how the Mahdi prevails in his Occultation, keeping in his possession the long recollection of what is, enriched by the anticipation of what will be, so well that the hope of it, pervaded by that total knowledge that is his alone, distinguishes itself from both the erratic or unfounded hopes common among mortals and the despair of people bound to a present that tortures them. The superiority of Nephite-Mahdite memory is forged in a consciousness that transits history as both actor in and testimony of history's permutations, turnings that depend on teaching and so suffer the vagaries of transmission or the discordant deformations to which the tradition is subjected by short-sighted individuals. In his *Preface to the Treatise on Vacuum*, Pascal, heralding the progress of science made by a "succession of men," considers "all the sequence of men over the course of the centuries . . . as one man who lives always and learns continually."[7] But Nephite-Mahdite time makes of humanity a man always having the first source present to his spirit.

One, then, is the time of the Messiah who appears suddenly in human time to entirely change its aspect. Another is messianic time that remains drawn out to this moment. And finally there is Nephite-Mahdite time, which introduces into the pulsation of human time a presence that endures and witnesses, the presence of a human being laboring and struggling, and not the presence of an institution, were it divinely established, or of a people, had it been set apart for the sanctification of the Holy Name. The differences are intrinsic.

Messianic time folds history in two: into the world (or age) of the here and now (*ʿolam hazeh*) and the world that comes (*ʿolam haba*).[8]

---

6. Cf. Muhammad Yaʿqūb al-Kulaynī, *Usūl al-kāfī* (Beirut: Dāt al-adwā, 1992), 1:298; Muhammad ibn Jarīr al-Tabarī, *Dalāʾil al-Imāmat* (Beirut: Al-aʿlamī, 1988), 30.

7. Blaise Pascal, *Thoughts, Letters, and Minor Works* (New York: Cosimo, 2007), 449.

8. Cf. Gérard Bensussan, *Le Temps messianique: Temps historique et tempe vécu* [Messianic time: Historical time and lived time] (Paris: Vrin, 2001), 8, 52–53. "The fold fractures the linear uniformity in what-there-is and what-comes. This stratification criss-crosses succession and superposition, contemporaneity and hope, instantaneity and patience. The fold constitutes an internal structuration of historical time, be it a

Nephite-Mahdite time knows and assumes the latter, but it offers its supplemental particularity to fold in two the world of the here and now—manifest and hidden.

What is the advantage of sempiternity? One gathers from various Imams that, since (and even before) Adam came to light, Allah has not left the earth without an Imam upon it—a condition for the Allah's worship-worthiness.[9] In contrast with the People of the Cave, who no longer count the nights,[10] those who are engaged with the care of the world keep watch and know. Rapture is not their concern. Such a figure hardly raises himself beyond the firmament when the world opens to his depths. Its thread must be preserved by coupling memory and hope, as does Orson Scott Card's Fiimma: "She sang to them as if she were as ancient as the Earth, as if all the pain of millennia of humanity had passed through her, leaving her scarred but whole, leaving her wise but hopeful."[11]

Since Mormon doctrine professes an extended period of apostasy running from the fifth to the nineteenth century, it would seem that God neglected humanity for an age. Thanks to the theory of the Three Nephites, that doctrine can redeem and justify itself in light of the teaching of President Joseph Fielding Smith. For since the beginning of and even during the apostasy, there was always someone in the sublunary region endowed with the priesthood to stand against Satan.[12] Therefore, Nephite-Mahdite time not only allows this person to tower over history, it also defines itself as a polemic. Its fold is that of opposition.

---

mobile and invisible disjunction: one never knows on which today the event folds itself" (translated from ibid., 158).

9. Ibn Bābūya, *Kamāl al-dīn wa-tamām al-niʿmah* (Beirut: Al-Aʿlamī, 2004), 199; "before, during, and after creation" (translated from ibid., 212). Cf. Muhammad Baqir al-Majlesi, *Bihār al-anwār* (Beirut: al-Wafāʾ, 1983), 52.92.

10. Cf. ʿAbd al-Karīm ibn Hawāzin al-Qushayrī, *Laṭāʾif al-ishārāt*, 6 vols., ed. Ibrāhīm Basyūnī (Cairo: Dār al-Kitāb al-ʿArabī liʾl-Ṭibāʿa waʾl Nashr, 1968), ad. 18:25.

11. Orson Scott Card, *Songmaster* (New York: Tor, 2002), 298.

12. Cf. Harold B. Lee, *Stand Ye in Holy Places: Selected Sermons and Writings* (Salt Lake City: Deseret Book, 1975), 161–62.

6

Lehi's Axiom

WHAT I CALL LEHI'S AXIOM is the first sentence and its corollaries in the following passage from the Book of Mormon: "It must needs be, that there is an opposition in all things. If [it were] not so . . . , righteousness could not be brought to pass, neither wickedness, neither holiness nor misery, neither good nor bad. Wherefore, all things must needs be a compound in one" (2 Nephi 2:11). It is by reason of this dynamizing opposition—a factor of the human liberty that acts only according to motives—that the Lord planted the two trees in Eden (see 2 Nephi 2:15–16). Thence, needless to say, proceeds the need for a devil. The prophet presents this deduction as his own: "And I, Lehi, according to the things which I have read, must needs suppose that an angel of God, according to that which is written, had fallen from heaven; wherefore, he became a devil, having sought that which was evil before God. And because he had fallen from heaven, and had become miserable forever, he sought also the misery of all mankind" (2 Nephi 2:17–18). The axiom is introduced as part of a reflection on the problem of retribution, joy, and punishment being equally necessary so that both law and creation might be (see 2 Nephi 2:10, 13).

On the basis of this axiom, Mormon author Bruce Dana seeks to corroborate the testimony of his coreligionist David Patten (one of Smith's first apostles; he died in 1838), who claimed to have twice encountered Cain, he who was condemned to wander for all time (although Mormon scripture itself barely supports such a theory). Just as the devil sets himself in opposition to the angel so that man's freedom is solidified by his being capable of good and evil, Cain will set himself head-on against John and the Three Nephites. His work—the work of him who forged an alliance with Satan (see Moses 5:30–31)—will be to consume souls, just as it will be John's work and the work of the Three Nephites to save them.[1] It is not enough to affirm, with Saint Augustine, that Cain is the founder of the earthly city.[2] Here, Cain has always accompanied Satan, seeking out those they might devour. The faculty of memory serves evil principles as well as good.

This allows me in turn to deduce that Nephite-Mahdite time itself is caught up in the schema of opposition, with or without the hypothesis of an anti–Three Nephites like Cain who would reproduce in human time the centuries-old antagonism between angels and demons—a conflict that becomes in Buddhism that of the Buddha (and the bodhisattvas) with Mara. The Mahdi must also conduct a decisive battle against the Dajjāl, the prince of lies, whom either the Mahdi or Jesus will slay.[3] Not surprisingly, this essential adversary who arises in the eschatological era is a man who must live through the ages, an idea from which Ibn Bābūya takes his argument in order to explain the longevity of the Mahdi.[4] The adversary is identified with a certain Ibn Säid (or Sayyād), who would have been a contemporary of Muhammad. The Dajjāl Messiah is widely understood to be the antagonist of the Messiah, son of Mary, in the Sunni tradition. The Dajjāl is, incidentally, seen in Jesus's wake in a dream of Muhammad.[5] Was he Jesus's shadow? A double? The

1. Bruce E. Dana, *The Three Nephites and Other Translated Beings* (Springville, UT: Cedar Fort, 2003), 108.

2. Augustine, *City of God* XV.1.

3. For an argument that Jesus will kill the Dajjāl, see Al-Asfahānī, *Muʿjam al-malāhim wa-l-fitan* (Tehran: n. p., 2002), 1:208, 228, 237–38. For arguments that it will be the Mahdi who slays the Dajjāl, see Ibn Bābūya, *Kamāl al-dīn wa-tamām al-niʿmah* (Beirut: Al-Aʿlamī, 2004), 477; and Muhammad Baqir Majlesi, *Bihār al-anwār* (Beirut: Al-Wafā', 1983), 52:194. For a suggestion that he will die by crucifixion, see ibid., 276.

4. Ibn Bābūya, *Kamāl al-dīn wa-tamām al-niʿmah*, 480–81.

5. See *Ṣaḥīḥ al-Bukhārī: The Translation of the Meanings of Ṣaḥiḥ al-Bukhari* (Riyadh: Darussalam, 1997), 60:48.

nocturnal element compounded in Jesus? In any case, this explains why he is made out to belong to the Jewish nation.[6]

Regarding his distinctive physical traits, one gathers that the Dajjāl is blind in one eye; among his powers is magic.[7] As for his morality, he is guilty of pride and deception, for he sought to pass himself off as a messenger of Allah and still proclaimed his own divinity.[8] He was a familiar of Muhammad, who saw through him in the daylight and asked Allah to take him away. He was therefore relegated to an island[9] until the hour of his eschatological reign, which will last forty years.[10] Here the application of Lehi's axiom is applied to astonishing effect: the need for equal, opposing forces ensures the progressive emergence of the idea that in response to the Mahdi's hidden physical presence another like presence must emerge. It is not enough, therefore, that an eschatological war against Sufiānī (whose name evokes the sworn enemy of Ali, the First Imam) summarizes every political conflict; what is needed is a centuries-long confrontation, however secret, in which two incarnate principles clash: good and evil.

Lehi's axiom is not unlike the theory of the Fifth Imam evoked above, according to which the faithful issue from a celestial substance, and thus infidels must stem from an infernal one. This radicalizes the antagonism between the two as if the infernal were a cause rather than an effect. A second dualism is created, as in the thought of Nasīr al-Dīn Tūsī, who sets in opposition to each other the followers of truth (*muḥiqqān*) and the followers of falsehood (*mubṭilān*).[11]

---

6. Al-Asfahānī, *Muʿjam al-malāhim wa-l-fitan*, 2:197.

7. Ibid., 2:208, 220. Here is a humorous detail: men were obliged to truss up their wives, daughters, and mothers in order to prevent them from following the Dajjāl (ibid., 2:231).

8. Ibid., 2:199, 205.

9. Ibid., 2:215. In this version, encountering him is possible if lost sailors wash up on his island (ibid., 2:214).

10. Ibid., 2:215.

11. Cf. Naṣīr al-Dīn al-Ṭūsī, *Paradise of Submission* §238. Note that this work is Ismaili.

There is still a path that leads to an ultimate profundity. The Tales of Alvin Maker, a series by Mormon novelist Orson Scott Card, gives this path a literary expression. He with whom Alvin, the character who embodies messianicity, must essentially cross swords is not the Devil as principle of moral evil but the enemy of all life, the Unmaker (or Uncreator, who is Non-doing and Non-being).[12] The Unmaker is a principle of ontological evil: that is to say, the power that can annihilate everything, dreaming of "undo[ing] the universe, break[ing] it all down until everything is flat and cold and smooth and dead"[13]—which is not true of the Devil, inasmuch as he cannot annihilate himself. In fact, the latter, like every man who destroys,[14] assists the former, but he does so without knowing it. The Devil would sooner ally himself with God than with the Unmaker in the great war.[15] But in this conflict, one does not see that evil involuntarily serves good, as Goethe's Mephistopheles must confess. The work of the Unmaker promotes no construction: "They always thought that Destruction was merely destruction, they were using it and when they were done with it, they'd set to building. But you don't build on a foundation of destruction. That's the dark secret of the Unmaker."[16]

Do we not run the risk here of letting these moments confront each other abstractly in an external relation? Put another way, do we not run the risk of failing to consider them as moments of life, which welcomes disjunction only when it serves the purposes of progress? It is the second corollary of Lehi's axiom that invites an admission of an internal link between the Unmaker and the Maker. Only in *The Crystal City* (volume 6 in the Tales) does Alvin imagine, without yet accepting it, that

---

12. Orson Scott Card, *Prentice Alvin* (New York: Tor, 1989), 96–98. The Unmaker corresponds in my thinking to Mephistopheles. Cf. Jad Hatem, *Satan, monothéiste absolu selon Goethe et Hallâj* [Satan: Absolute monotheist according to Goethe and Hallāj] (Paris: Éditions du Cygne, 2006). Alvin was the name of Joseph Smith's eldest brother (cf. D&C 137:5). Incidentally, Card's magical hero is a figuration of the Mormon Prophet and his successor.

13. Card, *Prentice Alvin*, 100.

14. Ibid., 97.

15. Orson Scott Card, *Seventh Son* (New York: Tor, 1987), 128.

16. Orson Scott Card, *Alvin Journeyman* (New York: Tor, 1996), 230–31.

destruction might play a role in construction, both belonging to "the same great flow of nature."[17] That seems to contradict the law evoked throughout Card's Tales according to which destruction advances faster than construction because, the deficit widening in favor of destruction, nothingness seems certain to extend its empire. And yet it does not, if one considers that the Maker does not face the Unmaker alone. The victory will finally belong to building up, thanks to the infinitesimal contributions of each: "And after a while, you come to realize that all those somethings, they add up to everything, and all the Unmaker's nothings, you put them all together and they're still nothing."[18]

Like the bodhisattva, Alvin, who "thinks he can save everybody,"[19] formulates a double vow: never to use his powers for personal gain[20] and to consecrate his entire life to the good of others, even if it be to construct and reinforce a reality in the face of the Unmaker's project of annihilation.[21] This certainly implicates the prohibition on killing,[22] a moral passivity, but also the obligation to fight. "Biggest of all [obligations is] to serve all men, and all lands," exclaims the red prophet Lolla-Wossiky,[23] a kind of shaman of nonviolence. Yet it is well understood that service requires confrontation.[24]

According to the first corollary of the axiom, the whole field of morality is polarized in the sense of a reciprocal dependence: without sin, we can do no good (see 2 Nephi 2:23). This corollary recalls the

17. Orson Scott Card, *The Crystal City* (New York: Tor, 2003), 221.

18. Ibid., 378–79. This notion is inscribed in an enumeration of acts that fall under ontology: building a family, a farm, etc. But ethics can be anchored there. Card says of the Unmaker that he "couldn't understand what Alvin was relying on: the power of decent men to act against their own interest in order to help those who trusted them." Orson Scott Card, *Heartfire* (New York: Tor, 1998), 248.

19. Card, *Heartfire*, 142.

20. Card, *Seventh Son*, 64.

21. Ibid., 166–67.

22. Orson Scott Card, *Red Prophet* (New York: Tor, 1988), 133.

23. Ibid., 185 (translator's addition).

24. Remarkably, the novel produces a wandering Jew—the condemned assassin Harrison—condemned to see his existence indefinitely prolonged without being able to shorten his days, so that he might tell and atone for his crimes.

fundamental law of opposition developed by the philosopher F. W. J. Schelling, which stipulates that no being can reveal itself except in its contrary: love in hate, unity in conflict, identity in difference.[25] Let us accord to this revelation an equally practical sense: one does not do good except in fighting evil; inversely, evil seeks to wound good.[26] As Joseph Smith puts it: "Wherever light shone, it stirred up darkness,"[27] which rings true, despite the paradox.

Because of the principle of sufficient reason (which wills that nothing be done without sufficient reason to determine why such a thing is rather than is not, and why it is the way it is and not another), this polarity cannot simply be a fact of nature; it responds to a finality. It was, in fact, decided on by God so as to galvanize human liberty (see 2 Nephi 2:15–16).[28] The first corollary does not offer an opinion on the substantial origin of opposition, which could only have been formally set down. Here we need the second corollary, which conceives a scission according to the principle of a vital activation by means of an internal contradiction (the yin and yang, for example, each containing the germ of the other). A compound in one is in principle susceptible to division and evolution, the core principle both of consciousness and life in romantic philosophy. So Schelling, tersely, asserts: "Without opposition no life, for man as for every existence in general."[29] Lehi seems to confirm this philosophy when he clarifies that "all things must needs be a compound in one; wherefore, if it should be one body it must needs remain as dead,

---

25. F. W. J. Schelling, *Philosophical Investigations into the Essence of Human Freedom*, trans. Jeff Love and Johannes Schmidt (Albany, NY: SUNY Press, 2000), 41, 129, 148.

26. Cf. Jad Hatem, *L'Echarde du mal dans la chair de Dieu* [The splinter of evil in God's flesh] (Paris: Cariscript, 1987), chapter 3, section 24.

27. Andrew F. Ehat and Lyndon W. Cook, eds., *The Words of Joseph Smith: The Contemporary Accounts of the Nauvoo Discourses of the Prophet Joseph* (Provo, UT: Religious Studies Center, Brigham Young University, 1980), 253.

28. This is echoed in a revelation attributed to Joseph Smith in September 1830: "And it must needs be that the devil should tempt the children of men, or they could not be agents unto themselves; for if they never should have bitter they could not know the sweet" (D&C 29:39).

29. Schelling, *Sämmtliche Werke*, 14 vols. (Stuttgart: Cotta, 1856–1861), 7:435.

having no life neither death, nor corruption nor incorruption, happiness nor misery, neither sense nor insensibility" (2 Nephi 2:11).

Through the emergence of divergent forces from an essential duplicity, the possibility of one overcoming the other is offered (which defines the power of good and evil). This dialectic may be explained as a case of a larger process: the overcoming of divergence itself. Schelling is careful to note that Nature hates division because division compels her to activity (whereas Nature aspires only to rest) and that she acts only to free herself of the obligation to act. But there attaches to her a fatality that her activity merely manages to revitalize the process of division: "The opposites must forever shun, in order forever to seek each other; and forever seek, in order never to find each other; it is only in *this* contradiction that the ground of all the activity of Nature lies."[30]

There remains to ask what the extension of the second corollary is. To be universal in its reach ("in all things"), does it envelop a reality superior to the angelic sphere? Might God be at once the Maker and the Unmaker, the Yea and the Nay? The Book of Mormon does not permit a judgment in favor of this supposition because all through 2 Nephi 2, God is completely distinguished from things (about which it is said that they comprise an opposition). However, a theological innovation of Joseph Smith more than a decade after the publication of the Book of Mormon invites us to submit divinity to the axiom and perhaps even to the second corollary. Whatever sense one is right to attribute to the later maxim, according to which God was not God for all eternity but at one time was a man like us,[31] it seems subject to the axiom and also to the corollary insofar as humanity, according to Smith, is the best place to progress, to pass "from grace to grace." This, the evidence suggests, we cannot do without overcoming and thus without the opposition comprised therein. All that becomes is always composed of and presupposes conflict, declared Aristotle.[32] But it is well understood, according to the

30. F. W. J. Schelling, *First Outline of a System of the Philosophy of Nature*, trans. Keith R. Peterson (Albany, NY: SUNY Press, 2004), 231.

31. Ehat and Cook, *Words of Joseph Smith*, 357.

32. See Aristotle, *Physics* 1.7 (189b30–191a23).

fundamental Schellingian law of opposition, that such becoming is accomplished as revelation. This is why Smith lets himself hope that one of his enemies, whom he qualifies as an adversary of truth, "will continue to stir up the sink of iniquity, that people may the more readily discern between the righteous and the wicked."[33] It seems that the imperative that adorns the axiom—"there must needs be . . ."—emanates from life itself: the lives of men, and the life of God; life that borrows its unique voice from the poetess:

> Hear how
> I open myself
> I am in every light.[34]

33. Joseph Smith Jr., "To the Elders of the Church of the Latter Day Saints," *Messenger and Advocate* (December 1835): 227.

34. Katarina Frostenson, *Canal*, trans. Christofer Bjurström (Beuvry: Maison de la poésie d'Amay, 1998), 73 (translated from the French).

By Way of Conclusion

A DISTANCE BETWEEN THE MYSTICAL and a religious messianic ethic aims to affirm the pure love one bears for God by postponing the blessedness envisaged eventually by the former. It is reported that when Christ asked John of the Cross what he desired in thanks for his service, the Saint replied, "Sufferings to be borne for Thy sake, and that I may be despised and counted as nothing."[1] One will note as well that messianicity is powerless to cover by itself the whole ethical field.

In the messianic ethic, being before men (*coram hominibus*) throws aside being-before-self (*coram meipso*) and being-before-the-world (*coram mundi*), and it is only if it has its place in a theistic religion that it doubles itself in being-before-God (*coram Deo*). But in exclusively occupying the center, being-before-men determines itself as being-for-men that ends in total self-sacrifice. One cannot hope to save one's place except by making the Unconditioned the standard by which to measure one's solicitude and philanthropy. It is only then that one will be able to adopt Goethe's proposition according to which "all conflict is eternal rest in God the Lord."[2]

The model of intelligibility I have attempted to elaborate across the discordances between the doctrines I have examined[3] inscribes in

1. Father Bruno of Jesus-Mary, *St. John of the Cross*, ed. Benedict Zimmerman (London: Sheed and Ward, 1932), xiv. John of the Cross was a sixteenth-century Spanish mystic.

2. J. W. von Goethe, *Selected Verse*, trans. David Luke (New York: Penguin, 1964), 280.

3. One can approach the idea of a messianic existential by means of theology. So it is that al-Ṣadr points out that the idea of the Mahdi is both older and further-reaching

history an immanent finality that, in order to fulfill the unfulfilled, takes human form. In this model, transcendence is not excluded, even for the bodhisattva. Immanence itself obeys a metahistorical tropism. It is not in this horizon that one pays the price to carry out the complete secularization of messianism. There is nothing particularly miraculous about human benevolence (though kindness is in itself excessive), but such benevolence does require a miracle—specifically, indefinite longevity—if it is to quench its vigilant passion while lodged in the heart of time. It is in the measure to which he is immeasurably free that the bodhisattva saves all others.[4]

than Islam, even if this particular religion expresses it better than all the others. Muḥammad Bāqir al-Ṣadr, *Bahth hawl al-Mahdī* (Qom: n.p., 1996), 55.

4. *The Flower Ornament Scripture* II.6.

Appendix 1

The Fundamental Law of Opposition: Lehi and Schelling

§ 1. Argument

In the chapter on evil (*Böse*, not *Übel*) of his work *The Theological Foundations of the Mormon Religion*, Sterling McMurrin considers what I have called Lehi's axiom, according to which there must necessarily be an opposition in all things (see 2 Nephi 2:11).[1] McMurrin offers two interpretations of the axiom. According to a first approach, evil exists to make good possible, which implies both that God creates or allows evil in the service of a greater good and that it is necessary to experience evil in order to appreciate the value of good (the latter of which implications McMurrin considers inappropriate). McMurrin prefers a second approach. Rather than stipulating that opposition must exist *purposively*, McMurrin is content to observe that opposition exists as a matter of fact, *inevitably*. Such a description would be confirmed by dialectical metaphysics (McMurrin mentions Taoism, Heraclitus, Hegel, and Marx) and cooperates with a theodicy founded on a reduction of God's power (God would not, under this option, have to produce or to allow evil).

I intend in this essay to defend a schema that combines the first option—interpreting Lehi's words in terms of the purposive existence

1. Sterling M. McMurrin, *The Theological Foundations of the Mormon Religion* (Salt Lake City: University of Utah Press, 1965), 97–98. Translator's note: *Böse* and *Übel* are German terms. They are different in the way that "evil" and "bad" are different in English. All *Böse* (evil) is *Übel* (bad), but not necessarily the reverse.

of evil—with a theme that belongs to the second option: the reduction of God's power, which guarantees his innocence. I exclude the idea that evil exists as a matter of fact. I do not agree with McMurrin that Hegel and Marx believed that evil inevitably exists, but I will not deal with such considerations here. My purpose is to implement Lehi's axiom, without removing it from its Mormon context, into a dynamic theodicy like that of F. W. J. Schelling. I have already—in chapter 6 of this book—linked Lehi's axiom with Schelling's fundamental law of opposition. Here I would like to compare Mormon theology with Schelling's *Philosophical Investigations into the Essence of Human Freedom* of 1809, where the law appears for the first time, so that I may draw the limits of the field where implementation would be justified. I will use the words *axiom* and *law* in order to distinguish formally Lehi's and Schelling's respective formulations.

I will start at the periphery, moving step by step toward the center, where I place the axiom and the law. I will then proceed with a comparison.

§ 2. Doctrinal Background

Mormon theology shares with Schelling's *Investigations* the latter's nonconformity with Christian orthodoxy. To whatever extent he was influenced by Luther, Schelling's conception of the nature of God and of his relationship with the world lies outside the frame drawn by Christianity. There is in Schelling no question of an Immanent Trinity since the Word is generated in view of the creation. Further, God is bestowed with a materiality in that his reason for being, rather than a simple notion (as in Leibniz), is consistent with a dynamic and desiring entity that will offer the universe its raw material. Finally, Schelling's God does not stand beyond time; he is becoming. These propositions are sufficient motives for comparison. Mormon theology, too, substitutes tritheism (or *at least* tritheism) for trinitarianism[2] and holds that God

2. See Orson Pratt, *The Essential Orson Pratt*, ed. David J. Whittaker (Salt Lake City: Signature Books, 1991), 380.

(or the gods)[3] is endowed with materiality and temporality. The *Natürphilosophie* that Schelling developed beginning in 1797 is all about acknowledging the consistency of the real as a foundation for the ideal. And Schelling's innovation in the *Investigations* is to think about God as both intratemporal and becoming. One can also say that Schelling's God is not simple since he is compounded with his "ground," which guarantees the personality "only" in which "is there life."[4] According to a well-known teaching of Mormon theology, God is composed of parts.[5]

The fact that God is not impassive and has human behaviors does not trouble either doctrine. Schelling claims a consequent anthropomorphism.[6] Mormon theology holds that God has a human form in the image of which man was created (see Ether 3:16) and even, according to a teaching traceable to Joseph Smith but not universally accepted, that he is himself of human origin.[7] Of the countless implications following from the idea of God's humanity, I will reflect merely that the connection between man and God is more than analogy: it is identity of structure, with a difference owed to God's own transformation. Joseph Smith accepts as literal the biblical assertion that Adam was created in God's

---

3. Abraham 4:1 passes in a single sentence from singular—"the Lord"—to plural—"and they, that is the Gods."

4. F. W. J. Schelling, *Philosophical Investigations into the Essence of Human Freedom*, trans. Jeff Love and Johannes Schmidt (Albany, NY: SUNY Press, 2006), 75. "God," says Schelling, "is the absolute unity of nature and personality." F. W. J. Schelling, *Philosophische Entwürfe und Tagebücher 1846: Philosophie der Mythologie und reinrationale Philosophie* (Hamburg: Meiner, 1998), 46.

5. See James E. Talmage, *Articles of Faith* (Salt Lake City: Deseret Book, 1982), 48; Pratt, *Essential Orson Pratt*, 79.

6. See Jad Hatem, *De l'Absolu à Dieu* [From the absolute to God] (Paris: Cariscript, 1987), chapter 2.

7. "God himself was once as we are now, and is an exalted man." Joseph Smith Jr., *History of the Church of Jesus Christ of Latter-day Saints*, ed. B. H. Roberts, 7 vols., 2nd ed. (Salt Lake City: Deseret Book, 1978), 6:305; from a discourse given by Joseph Smith on April 7, 1844, in Nauvoo, Illinois; reported by Wilford Woodruff, Willard Richards, Thomas Bullock, and William Clayton. Original transcriptions can be found in Andrew F. Ehat and Lyndon W. Cook, eds., *The Words of Joseph Smith: The Contemporary Accounts of the Nauvoo Discourses of the Prophet Joseph* (Provo, UT: Religious Studies Center, Brigham Young University, 1980), 340–62.

image. Unlike Druzism, Nuṣayrism, and even Orthodox Christianity, all of which require God to borrow human form in order to show himself to human beings (illusorily in the first two, actually in the third), Joseph Smith has no need for these expedients of religion, because even if Mormon theology allows for the Incarnation, it preserves God's power to manifest in human form independently of terrestrial flesh, since that form is proper to him. Thus it is that the Father appears to Joseph Smith.

Points of convergence with Schelling are as follows: man is ipseity and matter, like God. Both being spirit, they are solely distinguishable by the fact that the link between universal will and particular will is breakable in man—the condition for the possibility of evil—but is not so in God. They share a structure, then, but only in general, because there is one decisive difference: whereas Schelling's Absolute becomes progressively human, the Mormon God emerges from humanity.

Although I have used the word *creation* and will continue to do so, it is clear that Mormon theology and Schelling both disqualify an *ex nihilo* creation, which impacts the problem of theodicy since God cannot be held entirely responsible for what is or appears to be. Creation is, rather, a formation from a preexistent reality, totally distinct from the Demiurge according to Mormon theology and relatively distinct according to Schelling.

When it comes to the notion of being Almighty, things are more delicate, positions less certain. A knowledgeable Mormon like James E. Talmage can, based on the doctrine he holds and defends, affirm God's omnipotence.[8] However, McMurrin has a different opinion, demonstrable at once by his insistence that the Mormon God (who does not operate *ex nihilo*)[9] is not absolute, his further insistence that man's free will is assured, and finally by his analysis of the problem of theodicy, which deserves quotation here:

> Clearly the three concepts of the absolute goodness of God, the absoluteness of his power, and the positive reality of evil are not

8. See Talmage, *Articles of Faith*, 44.
9. McMurrin, *Theological Foundations of the Mormon Religion*, 27.

> mutually compatible as ingredients of a theistic world view. One of them must be compromised to save the other two. No cultured religion can sacrifice the first; traditional orthodox Christianity has at times lived with inconsistency and at other times hesitantly sacrificed the third; Mormonism, liberal Protestantism, and some philosophical theology have sacrificed the second.[10]

We ought to agree with McMurrin, who does not ignore Mormon theologians' and preachers' uses of the rhetoric of divine omnipotence but still holds that doctrine to be incompatible with the essence of Mormon theology.[11] Schelling's God is no less limited in his power. Although he uses for creation a material cause of which he is not the absolute master, he has not taken it out of nothingness, and he uses mankind (the good and the less good) to pursue the work of his own revelation. Hence the extraordinary lines: "Man stands on the threshold; whatever he chooses, it will be his act: but he cannot remain undecided because God must necessarily reveal himself and because nothing at all can remain ambiguous in creation."[12]

Among cases of divergence, ought we to mention pantheism? This seems obvious, insofar as Schelling claims he is a pantheist indeed, whereas according to Mormon theology the things that constitute the world are not modes of God. But besides the fact that this Spinozist characterization of pantheism, to which McMurrin assents,[13] is far from covering all forms of pantheism (it is certainly not that to which Schelling subscribes), the fact that the Mormon God is composed of matter (however subtle) leads, if not to pantheism as such, at least to a monist thesis—as in a universe that is substantially one—with the result that, however one might claim that the Mormon God is transcendent,[14] he is

10. Ibid., 105.

11. Ibid., 35. In his note about divine omnipotence in Daniel H. Ludlow, ed., *Encyclopedia of Mormonism*, 4 vols. (Macmillan: New York, 1992), David Paulsen specifies that this notion should not be taken in its traditional meaning of unlimited power, a contradictory concept.

12. Schelling, *Philosophical Investigations*, 41.

13. McMurrin, *Theological Foundations of the Mormon Religion*, 102.

14. Ibid., 9.

still made of the same substance as the rest of the universe. This is not obvious for Schelling. But then, McMurrin is totally mistaken when he brings together what he calls the transcendentality of Mormonism with Calvinism rather than with Lutheranism, which would rather agree with immanence. He ought, in fact, to have considered pagan theology, insofar as it (with the exception of neo-Platonism) conceives divinity (plural and singular) as intra-cosmic. At any rate, the rift between Mormon theology and Schelling's philosophy would not run between transcendence and immanence, but rather between monism (where God is *part* of everything) and theomonism (where God *is* everything).[15] We must specify that there are as many pantheisms as there are monisms. Some are reductive (spiritualist or materialist, for instance). Monism ought, in my opinion, to define the Mormon ontology that contains plurality. However, God's transcendence being relative, that ontology does not contradict Lévinas's definition of paganism as the "radical impotence to exit from the world. It does not consist in denying spirits and gods, but in placing them in the world" (or, if one prefers, in the immanence of the elements).[16] As enlarged as it can be, the world remains the world. The eternity of souls in Mormonism is of an elemental kind.

§ 3. Comparison

It is now possible to pursue a direct comparison between Lehi's axiom and Schelling's law of opposition. First, then, the texts.

1. What I call "Lehi's axiom" is a sentence attributed to the first great prophetic figure in the Book of Mormon—"For it must needs be, that there is an opposition in all things"—to

15. The monism of Mormonism—in its symmetry with pantheism—might be better called theo-in-panism. It should be noted that this aspect of Mormon doctrine appeared only eventually. The Book of Mormon itself inclines more to strict divine transcendence.

16. Emmanuel Lévinas, "L'Actualité de Maïmonide," *Cahier de L'Herne, Emmanuel Lévinas* (1991): 144.

which are appended first and second corollaries, as follows: "If not so, . . . righteousness could not be brought to pass, neither wickedness, neither holiness nor misery, neither good nor bad. Wherefore, all things must needs be a compound in one" (2 Nephi 2:11).

2. In the middle of his intellectual career, Schelling formulates his fundamental law of opposition in two different places: first in the *Philosophical Investigations into the Essence of Human Freedom* (1809) and second in the Stuttgart lectures (1810) that assign a name to the law.
    a. "Every essence can only reveal itself in its opposite, love only in hate, unity in conflict."[17]
    b. "*The fundamental law of opposition*. Without opposition no life, for man as for every existence in general."[18]

It is after the double announcement of the coming of the Messiah and of the necessity of a judgment that Lehi formulates his axiom. He must explain why judgment envelops punishment and happiness as opposites, judgment having to meet the requisites of atonement. Negating moral oppositions would lead to negating justice; it would be like denying God's existence. The book of Alma imagines this consequence in striking terms: if the work of justice could be destroyed, God would cease to be God (see Alma 42:13, 22, 25). Since God is the creator, according to Lehi, it is rather God who must put in question the existence of the world (see 2 Nephi 2:13). It is thus clear that Lehi is not content with acknowledging a stubborn, universal, moral, and cosmic or even theological fact (the inevitability of evil) because he presents it as an explanatory principle that gives meaning. That is, it *reveals*. It shows function but also *finality*. It is the necessary *condition* of things. The Doctrine and Covenants takes up the subject (and with more authority, as it reports what are held to be God's own words): "It must needs be

17. Schelling, *Philosophical Investigations*, 41.

18. F. W. J. Schelling, *Sämmtliche Werke*, 14 vols. (Stuttgart: Cotta, 1856–1861), 7:435.

that the devil should tempt the children of men, or they could not be agents unto themselves; for if they never should have bitter they could not know the sweet" (D&C 29:39).

Lehi's axiom is considered the condition, if not of freedom, at least of its practice. The bitter and the sweet evoke the two fruits of Eden and must be understood in a moral rather than in a physical sense since the mechanical passage from pain to pleasure and back to the pain that is the fate of human existence after the fall is not linked to any act of freedom. In ideational terms, what precedes evil is the fundamental law of opposition itself that guarantees freedom. Evil does not proceed from freedom. The latter is only the site of the emergence of evil.[19]

McMurrin thus takes the path of rational theodicy at the expense of the text's meaning when he chooses the explanation of opposition as a raw fact that would leave God safe from any imputation of evil. What is essential is not God but life, including divinity. Indeed, after the second corollary, Lehi specifies that if nothing were composite and all things were reducible to a single body, the divine would have neither life nor sensibility. I should note that when I say that divinity itself is submitted to oppositional polarity, I am alluding above all, in the immediate context, to the fall of the angel who becomes a demon because he sought for what was evil before God—an event reported by Lehi (see 2 Nephi 2:17). But I am *also* alluding to a Mormon teaching that follows closely the Book of Mormon, according to which Satan desired to be called Elohim's son by atoning for all of humanity. He demanded honor from God as his reward (see Moses 4:1), an honor considered in the Doctrine and Covenants as equivalent to divine power (see D&C 29:36).

It should be noted that, according to the just-mentioned account, Satan claims to suspend Lehi's axiom because of a desire to save all souls. This is subtly insinuated, since the text reports the Father saying that, in addition to rebelling against God, Satan was also trying to destroy man's agency (Moses 4:3). But opposition is, for Lehi, a condition of human

---

19. Neither Lehi nor Schelling would say, as does the Nusayri book *Kitab al-Haft wa-l-azillat* (chapter 6), that God created Satan out of the transgressions and sins of the believers.

freedom: "Wherefore, the Lord God gave unto man that he should act for himself. Wherefore, man could not act for himself save it should be that he was enticed by the one or the other" (2 Nephi 2:16). The two trees in paradise have become, here, symbols of a double postulate.

If there is irony in the Book of Moses account of Satan's rebellion, it is to be found in this unexpected project of Satan: instead of destroying opposition, he reinforces and figures it. He reinforces it by making tangible the contrast that was latent between Christ (the true Son, as the Father underscores) and Satan. And he figures it insofar as it is a secret opposition (first to the Father, but perhaps also to the Son) that encourages his candidacy. The power of reality is such that any maneuver must take it into consideration. Good cannot neglect the law of opposition out of idealism. Not only would it fail lamentably, it would also provoke in consequence a renewal of evil. The reverse is also clearly true: an excess of evil brings renewed good. Carl Jung gives this law the name of "enantiodromia," a running in the opposite direction.

However, this convocation of opposites maintains a mechanical and external character as long as the opposites are not revealed one in the other. Not only is one felt *by contrast with* the other, as with sour and sweet, but one comes *through* the other, which makes Schelling's intervention in this question so precious. I would thus distinguish four states of the law of opposition, starting with the least, as follows:

1. *The coexistence of contraries*. This consists in the simple fact that things are mixed. The idea is palpable in Lehi's discourse, but Giordano Bruno puts it into service: "Nothing is pure and simple. . . . All things consist of opposites, and thus the events that befall our emotions, because of the compounding that exists in things, cannot provide any enjoyment without some complement of bitterness."[20] We recognize in Bruno's words Lehi's axiom, as well as its second corollary, with the difference that for Lehi it is good and

20. Giordano Bruno, *On the Heroic Frenzies*, trans. Ingrid D. Rowland, ed. Eugenio Canone (Toronto: University of Toronto Press, 2013), 65.

necessary that things are submitted to compositeness—and that alters the entire perspective. For his part, Bruno prefers the middle region where the extremes cancel each other out.[21]

2. *The negative reciprocal determination of contraries.* Bruno goes on: "Indeed, I further declare and note that if there were no bitterness in things, there would be no enjoyment, because our exertions make us take pleasure in resting."[22] It is not by itself that a word is present to another, but by its absence, which connects to the linguistic theory of the zero degree. Bruno risks introducing the notion of causality: "[If we] examine matters in general, it will always be the case that one extreme provides the reason that its opposite becomes the object of longing and the source of pleasure."[23] But *this* law of contrasts only expresses a causality by default, against which the first corollary of Lehi's axiom inveighs, since it places the stakes at the level of morals and salvation in a way that implies freedom.
3. *The positive reciprocal determination of contraries.* Here causality is active and the law is truly dynamic. What is essential for Lehi is that the axiom ensures the basis for freedom. Without duality, there is no choice, and without duality of opposition, there is no ethical or religious choice, because there is only a choice of one term *against* another—something that Schelling conceived perfectly, since for him conflict is the main element of life and evil must be awakened in order to be overcome.[24] It is thanks to this polarity that the spark of life is communicated to the whole being. The second corollary redounds on the axiom and explains it, permitting its relocation from the first state of the law to the third state. But

21. See ibid., 69, 71.
22. Ibid., 65.
23. Ibid.
24. See Schelling, *Philosophical Investigations*, 63–64.

Schelling's theory includes an extra element, and thus it is advisable to consider a fourth state of the law of opposition.

4. *The positive reciprocal determination of contraries as a revelation of each.* Lehi supposes that good and evil are known, which causes some problems, since the boundary between them is blurry. First they must be defined, and then we need to be sure that one is not mistaken for the other. There are still more subtle confusions. We might correctly say that the better is the enemy of the good, and thus grant good two enemies: evil and that excess of good that very well might, out of an unwilling enantiodromy, call up the evil that it is not. A first conclusion, then, is that the apprehension of a reality implies the perfect knowledge of its contrary.[25]

Even if Schelling's thought touches on these issues, the essential point comes at an earlier stage and concerns the apparition of good and evil. Love requires hate as its opposite in order to be effective,[26] which amounts to saying that it remains latent without its opposite (*Gegenteil*). Indeed, love as a simple disposition is hardly more than impotence. That "hardly more" is, however, of high value because it is a lever, albeit at rest: a promise of fulfillment. For it to be fulfilled, it requires the element of conflict mentioned above—it must wrestle with hate. To appear (and appear here really means "to be"), it must win over an adverse force. Of course, the nature of hate complicates matters, since it is not inert, as if evil was a defect of good, a hole in being, the resistance of matter, or the end of an effort. Hatred must always oppose; it is not indifference. It searches for love in order to bring it down, and it would be timid if it did not find love, which is why it happens that evil can provoke good, not only after the fact (because of enantiodromy) but beforehand, in order to fulfill itself as evil, to achieve its highest degree. It is said that Gilles de

25. For example, "Only he who already knows his opposite through and through can look the spiritual right in the eye." F. W. J. Schelling, *Clara, or, On Nature's Connection to the Spirit World*, trans. Fiona Steinkamp (Albany, NY: SUNY Press, 2002), 28.

26. See Schelling, *Philosophical Investigations*, 41.

Rais, the greatest criminal of all time, imagined a scenario in which he would try to get his child victims to love him before he stabbed them.[27] Evil is the site of the revelation of good.

Schelling agrees with Lehi that there cannot be good or evil without opposition to justice or holiness. This assertion is sufficient in opening up space for freedom and retribution. But the philosopher goes further than the prophet in thinking that man's freedom is the act by which good and evil become what they are. For Schelling, freedom itself must begin by putting itself in its contrary (that is, necessity) in order to become efficient.[28]

Here is a second conclusion: what is at stake is not only a choice between two realities, but their coming into being. For opposites to be revealed *one in the other*, it is not enough to oppose indifference. Hatred, for instance, must be at its peak, its maximum of self-manifestation as hatred of love, if it is to be the very thing that must be vanquished by love. It is not without reason that Christ considers the sin against the Spirit as unatoneable. Indeed, this sin consists in declaring that the Man of Nazareth practices his healing gifts by the power of the devil. Is this not a claim that good is evil, and does this claim not thus seek to deliver a fatal blow to the good? It is, in any event, in this way that good and evil are at opposite ends of banality and must confront each other. This essential opposition is widely visible in the Book of Mormon, with no need for Lehi's axiom to underscore it.

In the blasphemous equation of good and evil ("good *is* evil"), the copula (*is*) may be understood in its *analytic* sense. The same equation can be found in Schelling's text, however, in order to express its *dialectical* value: to say that this *is* that is to say that this is the *foundation of* that. In other words, evil does not possess in itself the power of being.[29] But the philosopher only formulates the equation to express

27. See Jad Hatem, *L'Écharde du mal dans la chair de Dieu* [The splinter of evil in God's flesh] (Paris: Cariscript, 1987), chapter 3, section 7.

28. See the discussion in F. W. J. Schelling, *The Ages of the World*, trans. Jason M. Wirth (Albany, NY: SUNY Press, 2000). See also Schelling, *Clara*, 28.

29. See Schelling, *Philosophical Investigations*, 13.

the copula as such. The idea proper—that good is subject to evil—is of Thomist origin. Schelling uses the expression in a context particular to his thought when he claims that "good and evil are the same thing only seen from different sides, or evil is in itself, that is, considered in the root of its identity, the good, just as the good, to the contrary, considered in its turning from itself or non-identity, is evil."[30] Not that these two realities can be confused, of course, but they are only distinguished by their form. Good and evil combine differently the universal will and the particular will that are found in all things. In the good, universal prevails over particular, and the reverse pertains in evil, which makes of it a perversion rather than a privation of good. Instead of repeating that cold and heat may only be felt in contrast, Schelling claims something totally different. Cold can only be felt because the body is susceptible to opposites, and these opposites are composed of the same ingredients, the difference residing in their arrangement, even if this arrangement is determined by an element that comes from outside, the other root, which confirms that good is no less apt to fight than evil.[31]

§ 4. God and Opposition

When Lehi says that there must necessarily be an opposition in all things, he does not exclude anything or anyone. As God is submitted explicitly by Leibniz to the principle of sufficient reason, he is implicitly submitted by Lehi to the law of opposition. I have already evoked the opposition in divinity that emerges at the moment of the rivalry between Lucifer and Christ, which merely reflects the rivalry between the Father and the insidious candidate for the Father's divinity. The moment has arrived to demand a new argument.

Mormon doctrine claims the idea of God's mutability. But it cannot do without an internal and an external opposition. If I may intervene in a quarrel among Mormon theologians about whether God became

30. Ibid., 63–64.
31. Ibid. See also Plato, *Republic* 491e.

changeless or still depends on a dynamic perfection, I would say that Lehi's axiom encourages the second hypothesis. One can, of course, imagine many things about the nature of opposition *in* God (one might consider it to be sexual, for instance, as in the Kabbalah). But it would be best to ask Schelling, for whom God originates from the Groundless, which, being nondifference, does not allow for opposition as such but could still contain distinct principles that would only be opposed in their manifested state.[32] For example, Schelling regards evil as latent in the Absolute as a possibility, and it only arises into being to be eternally overcome. Latent good, moreover, only comes to be through overcoming, by which the opposed force that has been overcome is maintained as raw material.

I offer one example, taken from the Stuttgart lectures of 1810: God raises one of the principles that constitute him (selfishness) above another (love) such that creation becomes possible without endangering God's existence, since selfishness, which expresses ipseity, must be preserved.[33] If selfishness dominated love, God would be inverted, and rather than pantheism, pandemonism would have held sway! It is in this context that Schelling writes,

> For the ordinary, abstract mode of understanding, it seems surprising that God should contain a non-divine principle, without consciousness and lesser than him. To conceive God as an empty identity, however, is not to comprehend him at all. The necessity of this hypothesis can be proven by means of *the fundamental law of opposition*. Without opposition no life, for man as for every existence in general.[34]

The Absolute must itself go through separation and opposition so that life may make its shining appearance. But Schelling's God aspires throughout history to be all and to be in all, such that all oppositions

32. See Schelling, *Philosophical Investigations*, 68–69.
33. Schelling, *Sämmtliche Werke*, 7:439.
34. Ibid., 7:435.

are appeased.[35] If opposition is a fact of being, as Lehi claims, it is understandable that no fulfillment can put an end to it. If it is an element of revelation, as Schelling teaches, we can easily allow ourselves to hope that it will lose its acuity in proportion as the mystery is elucidated—that is to say, that love will reign. "The non-ground divides itself into the two exactly equal beginnings, only so that the two, which could not exist simultaneously or be one in it as the non-ground, become one through love, that is, it divides itself only so that there may be life and love and personal existence."[36] We understand that hatred must first be made manifest. But God is not directly capable of the power of good and evil: a relative impotence of God, but oh so reassuring!

On scission and the hope for union, the young Schelling of his *First Outline of a System of the Philosophy of Nature* wrote some inspired lines. Although they concern Nature, I dare to believe that they are also applicable to God and to the fundamental law of opposition:

> Nature is the *laziest of animals* and curses separation because it imposes upon it the necessity of activity; Nature is active only in order to rid itself of this compulsion. The opposites must forever shun, in order forever to seek each other; and forever seek, in order never to find each other; it is only in *this* contradiction that the ground of all the activity of Nature lies.[37]

---

35. See Schelling, *Philosophical Investigations*, 70.

36. Ibid.

37. F. W. J. Schelling, *First Outline of a System of the Philosophy of Nature*, trans. Keith R. Peterson (Albany, NY: SUNY Press, 2004), 231.

Appendix 2

Yahweh Is Jesus

§ 1.

Because several names are proposed for the biblical God—certain of them acknowledged as proper names, others as common names—the temptation is strong to correlate divinity to qualities, to hypostases, and even to distinct entities. In tracing the word *divinity*, I prepare in this essay the possibility of a way out of strict monotheism.

As an example, the precious Gnostic document entitled the *Apocryphon of John* recounts that Yaldabaoth fathered two sons by Eve: the bear-faced Yahweh and the cat-faced Elohim—the first unjust and the second just—better known by the names Abel and Cain.[1] One will note that the two divine names designate different personages with the nature of Gnostic archons (which, according to the Gnostics, does not ultimately distinguish these personages from the Old Testament demiurge) and that their respective value is inverted in relation to the text of Genesis: the performer of the bloodless sacrifice is preferred over his brother. But fairness does not confer the grace of goodness.

In the pages that follow, I propose to analyze two traditions inspired by Christian gnosis that confer upon Jesus the name of Yahweh to the exclusion of the Father.

1. See James M. Robinson, *The Nag Hammadi Library*, rev. ed. (San Francisco: HarperCollins, 1988), 118–19.

§ 2.

Certain exegetes, the Mormons among them,[2] derive the proper name Yahweh, the causative form of the imperfect tense of the Hebrew verb *hawah* (to become), from *Ehyeh* (*I Am*), which comes from the self-revelation of God to Moses: "I Am that I Am" (Exodus 3:14). The Mormons use this derivation to identify Yahweh with Jesus Christ on the basis of two things: (1) the fact that the latter pronounces "I am" in the New Testament (John 8:58) and then makes a name of the phrase in their own unique scriptures: "Listen to the voice of Jesus Christ, your Redeemer, the Great I Am, whose arm of mercy hath atoned for your sins" (D&C 29:1); (2) the significance of his name—Yehoshua: literally, *Yahweh saves*—so that it would be him who, master of the work of sacred history, both gave the law to Moses (see 3 Nephi 15:5) and then took upon him flesh: "the God of Abraham, and of Isaac, and the God of Jacob, yieldeth himself, according to the words of the angel, as a man" (1 Nephi 19:10). Thus James E. Talmage comments:

> Jesus of Nazareth, who in solemn testimony to the Jews declared Himself the *I Am* or *Jehovah*, who was God before Abraham lived on earth, was the same Being who is repeatedly proclaimed as the God who made covenant with Abraham, Isaac, and Jacob; the God who led Israel from the bondage of Egypt to the freedom of the promised land, the one and only God known by revelation to the Hebrew prophets.[3]

Talmage's formulation "the one and only God" here does not serve the proponent of monotheism. It serves, rather, to exclude God the Father from candidacy for the title of Yahweh (even though the canonical Mormon books hardly invite this exclusion)[4]—not that the Father has

---

2. See, for example, James E. Talmage, *Jesus the Christ: A Study of the Messiah and His Mission according to Holy Scriptures Both Ancient and Modern* (Salt Lake City: The Deseret News, 1915).

3. Ibid., 38.

4. For instance, it is more probable that, considering context, it is to the Heavenly Father that the name Jehovah is attributed throughout section 109 of the Doctrine and Covenants.

no role to play, but he confines himself to attesting to the dignity of his Son and inviting people to listen to him (see 3 Nephi 11:7). When it is professed in the Book of Mormon that "there is one God and one Shepherd over all the earth" (1 Nephi 13:41), it is helpful to understand that this refers exclusively to the Son. While John's prologue makes the Only Begotten the instrument of the inaugural act, Mormon scripture—in spite of the Nicene Creed—attributes the creation to the Son exclusively: "My hand hath also laid the foundation of the earth, and my right hand hath spanned the heavens. I call unto them and they stand up together" (1 Nephi 20:13). The Son thus inherits in Mormonism attributes that the patristic tradition confers foremost on the Father: *omnipotens, omnicreans, omnitenens*.[5] It is notable that, in general, the Book of Mormon rarely departs from the standard practice of translating the Tetragrammaton (the four sacred letters lying behind the voiced name Jehovah) as "Lord."[6] The use of Jehovah becomes somewhat more commonplace in the Doctrine and Covenants. In the Pearl of Great Price, the Lord ("the Lord my God") gives himself the name Jehovah (see Abraham 1:16).

A Book of Mormon passage that declares that Christ is both Father *and* Son is problematic, even for the Mormons. According to the text, he is "the Father, because he was conceived by the power of God; and the Son, because of the flesh" (Mosiah 15:2–3; cf. Ether 3:14). The official explanation for this is layered: Christ is the Father (1) inasmuch as he is the creator of all things, (2) by virtue of his sacrifice for those who recognize it, and (3) because of the investiture he receives from his Father.[7]

The name Elohim, absent from the Book of Mormon, is one Mormons eventually reserved for the Father, of whom Yahweh is the firstborn son.[8] But before this relatively late and unexpected development in Mormon teaching, *elohim* was used as a common name or predicate by the religion's

5. See Augustine, *The Literal Meaning of Genesis* IV.12; Augustine, *Confessions* 11.3–8.

6. For examples, see 2 Nephi 22:2 and Moroni 10:34, the last verse in the book.

7. This is clarified in a well-known declaration made by the First Presidency on June 30, 1916. See James E. Talmage, *Articles of Faith* (Salt Lake City: Deseret Book, 1982), 466–67.

8. Ibid., 472.

founder, Joseph Smith, who, discovering that the word is a Hebrew plural, hastened to make further use of it in professing polytheism.[9]

We observe, then, that the Mormon exegetes take, so to speak, the path opposite that of the redactors of the Pentateuch—who belonged to two different parties aligning with two distinct theologies, so much so that the Yahweh of the Yahwist barely resembles the Elohim of the Elohist and the Priestly Code. The redactors of the books attributed to Moses produced a harmonization, such that in the end the two names Yahweh and Elohim could be associated (as in the Hebrew of Genesis 2:7, for example), and the same sequence could make them succeed each other—it being well understood, in the spirit of the common reader, that the referent of the terms remains the same.

§ 3.

But what is the goal of the Mormon distribution of divine names? And is it likely to determine the specificity of the Son?

The first answer to come to mind is that the distinction between Elohim and Yahweh supports an anti-Trinitarian argument. In effect, for traditional Christianity, Elohim is the common name of three hypostases. (Even better, it is a plural controlling a singular verb.) Even if the Holy Name is often attributed to the Father, it is equally valid when applied to the Trinity, and thus to the Son. As in John Donne's writings, Christ may at times be distinguished from Yahweh, the latter taken as equivalent to Being,[10] but this gesture is exceptional. On the other hand, it is not rare to see the Tetragrammaton engraved in the frescoes

---

9. See Andrew F. Ehat and Lyndon W. Cook, eds., *The Words of Joseph Smith: The Contemporary Accounts of the Nauvoo Discourses of the Prophet Joseph* (Provo, UT: Religious Studies Center, Brigham Young University, 1980), 379. In the Pearl of Great Price, the "gods" organize the world (see Abraham 4).

10. "Man in general hath relation to God, as he is Jehovah, Being; we have relation to Christ, as he is Jesus, our salvation; salvation is our being, Jesus is our Jehovah." John Donne, *The Works of John Donne*, 6 vols. (London: John W. Parker, 1839), 2:383–84 (Sermon 48, on Psalm 6:1).

representing Christ as a testament to his divinity and his consubstantiality with the Father, which justifies one in saying that it is Christ the Lord who led Israel out of Egypt.[11]

Now, if the Mormons confess the divinity of the Son (whatever their concept of divinity is at the moment), they reject consubstantiality—in consequence of which one finds before one a divine triad rather than a divine trinity. It is interesting to note that another theory that distances itself from Trinitarian dogma, namely the Arianism of Jehovah's Witnesses, has taken the opposite tack to Mormonism, seeing it confers the name Yahweh uniquely on the Father because it does not consider the Son identical to or of the same nature as the Father (i.e., the Uncreated). One is led, therefore, to an original configuration when one reads in Mormon writings that Yahweh is Jesus, and *not the Father*.

I said just now that in the mind of the common reader of the Pentateuch, the referent remains the same whether one says "Elohim" or "Yahweh." But the common reader is hardly the only reader. In the Kabbalah, the two names refer back to different Sephirot—which, while being distinct entities, are no less than expressions of the one Deity (the Infinite) deployed in ten ways that are at once centered on themselves and communicative of themselves to others. In this layered deployment of the Deity, Yahweh correlates primarily to the Sephira Tipheret,[12] whereas the name of Elohim fits in the same way with the Sephira Malkuth.[13] The two Sephirot illustrate the particularity of being called to couple as masculine and feminine (or sun and moon).[14] This is to say that they constitute a sort of dyad at the heart of the decad. As it is Elohim who governs the earth, he is perforce known by all peoples,

11. This is the case of Assemani, even though he does not evoke the work *ad extra* of the Trinity. See Giuseppe Simone Assemani, *Kitab al-Ilahiyyat* (Zouk Mosbeh: Notre Dame University–Louaize Press, 2003), 1059.

12. See *Zohar* 1.150b. To be more specific: primarily because Yahweh can represent all the Sephirot, since he is at the center of everything, he can assure their coalescence (see ibid., 193b). Among the patriarchs, it is Jacob who represents Tipheret.

13. See ibid., 1.22a, 1.144b, 1.150b.

14. See ibid., 1.144b.

but that is not so in the case of Yahweh, reserved for Israel, who manifests himself in mercy only when the righteous are found in the world.[15]

The remarkable thing about this, if one were to propose a quick comparison between Kabbalah and Mormonism, is that Elohim takes second position in the *Zohar*, whereas he is first in Mormon thought.[16] In both cases, Yahweh is called Son,[17] but in the Kabbalah this is for the simple reason that he issues from greater Sephirot. We retrieve from this analysis the idea that the two divine names are dissociable in the two traditions—Mormonism and Kabbalah. But there is a way to go forward by having recourse to Christian Kabbalah, which, taking license from the Zoharic, proceeds to the same disjunction and above all confers on Jesus the title of Yahweh exclusive of the Father.

The initiator of this gesture is Pico della Mirandola, who, in his *Conclusions*, announces: "The three great four-letter names of God, which exist in the secrets of the Cabalists, through miraculous appropriation should be attributed to the three Persons of the Trinity like this: so that the name *Ehyeh* is that of the Father, the name YHVH of the Son, the name Adonai of the Holy Spirit."[18] To the Father, therefore, goes the seminal name Ehyeh; to the son, Yahweh, the name derivative of the seminal one; and to the Spirit, Adonai, lordship. Now the name of Yahweh, since it befits the Son, must equally be applied to the Christ: "By the name *Yod he vav he*, which is the ineffable name that the Cabalists say will be the name of the Messiah,[19] it is clearly known that he will be God the Son of God made man through the Holy Spirit."[20]

---

15. See ibid., 1.195a.

16. This is often understood differently when Elohim is identified with Gevurah, as in Moses de Léon, *Le Sicle du sanctuaire* [The Shekel of the Sanctuary], trans. Ch. Mopsik (Lagrasse: Verdier, 1996), 284.

17. See *Zohar* 1.124b.

18. Giovanni Pico della Mirandola, *Syncretism in the West: Pico's 900 Theses (1486): The Evolution of Traditional Religious and Philosophical Systems*, ed. Stephen A. Farmer (Tempe, AZ: Medieval and Renaissance Texts and Studies, 1998), 523.

19. Cf. Babylonian Talmud *Baba Batra* 75v.

20. Pico della Mirandola, *Conclusions*, 527.

Two of the letters (composing, incidentally, the Tetragrammaton) play a particular role, for Pico, in the conception of the human nature of the Savior: "Through the mystery of the two letters *vav* and *yod*, it is known in what way the Messiah as God was the beginning of himself as man."[21] Regarding the seminal name, we note that the Kabbalists of the ʿIyyun group maintain that the true name of God, he who is the source of EHYH and YHVH, is EHVY.[22] In this way, they ascend towards the abyss of the origin of the deity.[23]

It is remarkable that Pico, instead of explicitly identifying the Trinity with the three greater Sephirot—Keter, Chokhmah, and Binah, those which Kabbalah itself exalts—chose to arrange the whole group in a sephirotic tree. In effect, Ehyeh traditionally designates the Sephira Keter,[24] the chiefest of the Sephirot. YHVH Tipheret occupies the middle of the tree, running between the Hebrew letter *he* above (Binah) and the letter *he* below (Malkuth).[25] As for Adonai, it refers to the Sephira Malkuth.[26] The *Zohar* eventually reunites these three names, but with a fourth, Tsevaot, applied to the Sephira Yessod,[27] whose nature it is to bring together all the Sephirot of the central column in whom the left and the right find equilibrium and who, in and beginning with Tipheret, ponders Strictness with Mercy.

If one insists on the messianic idea, Tipheret gains importance and monopolizes all divine substance, as happens with the Messiah Sabbatai

21. Ibid., 539.

22. Cf. Gershom Scholem, *Le Nom et les symboles de Dieu dans la mystique juive* [The name and symbols of God in Jewish mysticism], trans. M. Hayoun and G. Vajda (Paris: Cerf, 1983), 79.

23. Translator's note: This is a paradox Hatem invoked in his discussion about the various messianic figures who increase in virtue and enlightenment only to descend further into the depths of the human condition to help those whose suffering or sinfulness is most abject and profound.

24. For example, Moses de Léon, *Le Sicle du sanctuaire*, 278–80. Sometimes Binah or Chokhmah.

25. See *Le Zohar, Cantique des cantiques* [The Zohar: Song of Songs], trans. Ch. Mopsik (Lagrasse: Verdier, 1999), 59.

26. See ibid., 286.

27. *Zohar* 2.61d.

Zevi, except Zevi dared not identify himself with divinity but by an ascendant participation in it (a movement in the opposite direction to that of the Word, who takes on flesh). Johann Reuchlin, who also considers the ineffable Name proper to the Messiah,[28] inserts into the sacred Name the Hebrew letter *shin*, which is supposed to render the name of Jesus as Messiah—YHShVH—all to insist on his relationship to Mercy.[29]

In conclusion, if we agree that the Yahweh of the Kabbalah casts light on the Mormon Yahweh, it would appear that, besides the messianic character discussed throughout the book to which this essay is appended, he possesses the attributes of peace and truth, which are, according to the *Bahir*, the fundamental traits of the sixth Sephira. We add to them the coalescing power, but not the equilibrium of contrasting positions, because the Mormon Yahweh aligns with the paternal will in emphasizing his opposition to the will of Lucifer, who serves as antagonist, and for this he does not synthesize being in reconciling that will with himself.[30] It must not be forgotten that *Tipheret* means "beauty," and thus "harmony." The Mormon Yahweh aims for the heights through opposition, whereas the Zoharic Yahweh unifies in his breast the contraries that the divinity knew to put in place.

---

28. See Johann Reuchlin, *On the Art of the Kabbalah*, trans. Martin and Sarah Goodman (Lincoln, NE: University of Nebraska Press, 1993), 113.

29. See ibid., xix. *Zohar* 1.100b proposes its own nominative fusion between YHVH and ADNY for the good reason that the second is the qere of the first, which gives YAHDVNHY.

30. See appendix 1, "The Fundamental Law of Opposition: Lehi and Schelling."

Appendix 3

Interview with Jad Hatem

James E. Faulconer

In April 2014 I sent Jad Hatem a series of questions about his book Postponing Heaven, *hoping he might say something about the origin of the book and also that our discussion might tease out some of its implications. Hatem's responses were thoughtful and informative, not only relating how he came to write* Postponing Heaven, *but also comparing Jesus Christ's work with the work of the bodhisattva and saying more about what he means by "Nephite-Mahdite time." Even more important, Hatem explains why he believes that the story of the Three Nephites is more central to the Book of Mormon and perhaps to Mormon self-understanding than scholars of Mormonism have previously recognized.*

—James E. Faulconer

James E. Faulconer: American readers will be surprised to find that a Lebanese philosopher has written a book that deals with not only Islam and Buddhism, but Mormonism. Can you tell us how this book came about?

Jad Hatem: The book is a result of a passion and a circumstance. I have a passion for religions in general, each of which I take to embody the attempt to decipher the mystery of human being in terms of its animating transcendent dimension. The circumstance was a course I gave in 2007 on Mormon doctrine. The course made me discover the point of contact between Mormonism, Buddhism, and Shiʿite Islam. That gradually suggested the possibility of writing a short book combining the philosophical point of view (implementing the transcendental of messianicity) and the point of view of the academic study of religions, without neglecting the literary dimension—since I did a fair bit of work on the novels of Orson Scott Card to support my argument.

As for the two essays appended to the main work: During my stay at BYU in 2008, at your invitation, I had the opportunity to take part in the meetings of the Society for Mormon Philosophy and Theology that took place that year at the University of Utah. I took that opportunity to develop the theme of chapter 6 of this book, "Lehi's Axiom," through a confrontation with Schelling. I am among those who believe in the virtue of comparison.

The idea of the second essay came to me while reading Pico della Mirandola: I brought together two distant stars. Needless to say, through that meditation I found a way of satisfying my passion for Christology. I would add that I have also published a comparative study of Catholicism and Mormonism on the question of Christ's will in Gethsemane (in my *Les Agonies du Christ* [Éditions du Cygne, 2010], chapter 2).

JEF: I notice that your book is dedicated to someone who is a Latter-day Saint leader in Lebanon, Karim Assouad. Can you tell us something about your reasons for that dedication?

JH: When I began work on the article that eventually developed into this book, I was short on resources. I had only read the Book of Mormon. I asked my students if any of them knew of a member of the Church of Jesus Christ of Latter-day Saints living in Lebanon. One of them gave me the telephone number of a local Mormon leader. That same day, I met him and obtained the Pearl of Great Price and a copy of the Doctrine and Covenants. Then he lent me the entire seven-volume *History of the Church*. A sense of fellow-feeling developed between us then and strengthened over time to become a genuine friendship.

Therefore it seemed natural for me to dedicate the book to him. And I must attribute the fact that he tirelessly tries to convert me to his faith to his good feelings toward me.

JEF: In your book you suggest that the writing of the Book of Mormon probably began with 3 Nephi. Can you explain more fully your reasoning for that conclusion? Is that assumption important to your understanding of the Book of Mormon? If so, how?

JH: The hypothesis to which you refer is based on my belief that the central kernel of the Book of Mormon is ethico-soteric in character and not, for example, mystic. What 3 Nephi highlights is the desire to devote one's life (prolonged or not) to the salvation of others. The spiritual experiences reported by Joseph Smith as visual and aural revelation seem to me to be oriented toward that mission.

JEF: Royal Skousen's critical text project (which only came to fruition after your book was published) has made reasonably clear that Joseph Smith and Oliver Cowdery began their work on the Book of Mormon with what is now the book of Mosiah. How does that development in Book of Mormon research change (or not) your thoughts on this issue? Is it possible to see all of the section from Mosiah through 3 Nephi as anticipating and working toward the ethico-soteriological concerns of 3 Nephi?

JH: There are good reasons to grant the book of Mosiah primacy insofar as it refers to the brass plates written in Egyptian, plates whose reading is necessary to safeguard the discourse (see Mosiah 1:2–5). Speaking as a nonbeliever, I see that as a good starting point for Joseph Smith, who needed to convey a similar conviction to his contemporaries. In proposing in my book that 3 Nephi was the starting point for Joseph Smith's dictations of the Book of Mormon, my judgment obviously proceeded not from philological analysis, but from an intuition that didn't get much beyond intuition. That intuition definitely lay in how I understood Joseph Smith's state of mind when he embarked on his project. I find it difficult to imagine that it was not part of Joseph Smith's idea from the outset to ground his own version of sacred history in a parallel manifestation of Christ (on American soil).

JEF: You say that the Three Nephites are "the three mysterious pillars upon which the church is built." Is that a comment about the LDS Church and contemporary Mormonism? Does the story of the Three Nephites and your analysis of that story suggest anything about Mormon self-understanding, not just what it is, but what it might or should be?

JH: All I can say is that the approach usually taken toward the story of the Three Nephites has been folkloric, and I felt that, instead, the episode deserved to be considered philosophically.

JEF: You say "the bodhisattva [exerts himself] in order to be able to share what he accumulates, the Christ in sharing what he has already won." How do the terms *in-place-of-others* and *beneath-others* apply to the work of the bodhisattva and that of Christ? Are they in tension? How do those terms apply to the work of the Three Nephites?

JH: Rather than tension, the relation is that of complementarity between two types of substitution (beneath-others, in-place-of-others). What is essential to the Three Nephites, the bodhisattva, and the Mahdi is precisely that they cannot fulfill their mission by *dying* for others. If they sacrifice their own existence, it is only by consecrating it. In their eyes the world remains present even if sometimes terribly so. Thus they are not examples of Paul Celan's very beautiful line—"The world is no more, I must carry you" (*Die Welt ist fort, ich muß dich tragen*). Nonetheless they connect with that poetic line by their phoric gesture (the fact of carrying, of being pillars). The Three Nephites do not imitate Christ by dying for others since, precisely, they are *preserved* in order to come to the aid of humanity—that aid is the work of conversion no doubt, but also, if one is to believe the folklore, of punctual interventions to help out this or that person.

JEF: It is not unusual for Mormon intellectuals to be attracted by the metaphysics of Buddhism. But your understanding of the Three Nephites puts them in contrast with the bodhisattva. Does that suggest that the attraction of Buddhism for some Mormons may include a misunderstanding?

JH: It seems to me that the Buddhism that attracts Mormons is probably that of the Lesser Vehicle (Hīnayāna Buddhism), which is more strictly materialist, metaphysically. It is clear that what I have mobilized in my study is the Buddhism of the Greater Vehicle (Mahāyāna Buddhism), which admits the immateriality of essence. And in any case, the point of convergence that I have underscored pertains to the ethical, rather than the metaphysical, sphere.

JEF: This is one of my favorite quotations in your book:

> Put another way, in Christianity human fulness models itself after the divine fulness of the second hypostasis of the Trinity; in Mahāyāna Buddhism, hypostasis must first dissolve itself so that the "I" can become all others. But precisely because of this emptiness, this last gesture is in everyone's reach, while because of the divine (and indissoluble) fulness of the second hypostasis, the Christian act is unique. The Three Nephites naturally dwell below these figures because neither their ontological constitution nor their vocation authorizes them to attend to humanity except nominally, for their Messiah is already doing it effectively.

Can you say anything more about this observation? What, for example, does this suggest about someone like Joseph Smith, who presumably had contemporaneous experience with the Three Nephites and was certainly contemporaneous with Mormon and Moroni, who were ministered to by the Three Nephites? What might it say for the contemporaneity of today's Latter-day Saints?

JH: I might summarize the point of the lines you quote as follows: the Three Nephites have the power neither to save the world (something already accomplished anyway) nor to annihilate their egos in order to be able to substitute themselves for all others indiscriminately.

That said, it is difficult for me to respond to the second part of your question, that about Joseph Smith. Did he meet our three persons? One must be a Mormon (1) to suppose the existence of the Three Nephites (and all other Nephites and Lamanites) and, so, (2) to admit the possibility of such meetings. The question of contemporaneity is nevertheless essential in a phenomenological approach to the consciousness of being Mormon. I explain in this book why Joseph Smith, being a prophet, did not need to personally experience contemporaneousness with Christ through the mediation of the Three Nephites. In spite of that, the faithful could feel (and have felt) that such an encounter was necessary.

This is also primarily a question of testimony: I can see and hear those who have seen and heard. We understand the importance of this when we remember that the faith of the Christian tradition as a whole depends entirely on the testimonies of women and men who witnessed the resurrection of Christ.

JEF: Another of my favorite quotations:

> The contemporaneity of the Three Nephites cannot ignore eschatological expectation, for their duration unravels a time-for-others charged with guaranteeing the continuation of history. The future dwells in coming. What mediates between worlds is the creative synthesis of the promise and of time (itself a combination of spirit and of world) such that history has at its immanent center a purely human standard-bearer.

Can you say more about your claim?

JH: It is not enough to *be* the contemporary of a contemporary. One must also *become* such—in other words, to become aware of it as a task. Mormons must think that the Three Nephites can be imitated so as to make more likely the possibility of choosing between the two forms of substitution discussed before. But if we look more precisely at their ontological (rather than ethical) specificity, we see that specificity (namely, their prolonged temporality) as a living bridge thrown between the original Christian revelation and the "latter days" in which Mormonism arises. Insofar as Mormonism accuses the Christian tradition of apostasy (that is, of a long rupture with the truth), it ought to be grateful to the Three Nephites (and the Apostle John) for preserving continuity.

JEF: What is the theological significance of the occultation of holy people—the *nistar*, the Mahdi, the Three Nephites? You say that continual presence would mean that "a theology of presence would have prevailed over a theology of hope," but what gives the theology of hope a positive valence in comparison to a theology of presence?

JH: A theology of presence deprives human beings of their liberty if God manifests himself as such in person, that is to say, by imposing himself in the full revelation of what he is. In that case, everything has been done, and the mortal person would have no other choice than to recognize and to obey him absolutely. But if a man of God shows himself as such, people are only partially deprived of their liberty because they continue to have room for faith. A person might not recognize the validity of the testimony of the prophet (or Messiah, etc.). Furthermore, not everything has been done. Time has not been entirely unfolded, ensuring that there is room for mystery, waiting, struggle, and hope.

JEF: You note that Joseph Smith put into place a system that safeguards prophecy from one president to the next rather than a system that would have allowed the occulted Three Nephites to act through a deputy. That, you say, explains the church's present structure. But don't you think that would also suggest a preference for theological reflection rather than personal revelation? Yet the LDS Church continues to emphasize direct encounter with the supratemporal at the same time that it safeguards the position of the Prophet.

JH: Of course I am no specialist in Mormon theology. But perhaps you are right. If so, then that suggests that there is a tension in Mormon history between the two kinds of contemporaneity. The institution wins out over anarchic shifts, certainly. But it runs alongside a popular belief in direct encounters with mediating angels.

JEF: You say, "And finally there is Nephite-Mahdite time, which introduces into the pulsation of human time a presence that endures and witnesses, the presence of a human being laboring and struggling, and not the presence of an institution, were it divinely established, or of a people, had it been set apart for the sanctification of the Holy Name." You are reasonably well acquainted with the Latter-day Saints. To what degree do you think that the fold of messianic time and its assumption of Nephite-Mahdite time is effective in present Latter-day Saint religious practice? To what degree do you think it is in danger of being overtaken by secular or some other time?

JH: The caveat I offered to the previous question applies equally well here. Given what I've already said about the possibility of a tension between two kinds of contemporaneity in Mormonism, perhaps the institution of the church or the people of the church has exactly replaced the Nephite-Mahdite experience of time. In that case, the sublation of the two kinds of contemporaneity by merely secular or secularizing time may have already occurred or be occurring. Like most other people, many Mormons are understandably skeptical of the folklore stories of the Three Nephites. Miracles seem impossible, especially when they deal with such things as flat tires. The longevity ascribed to the Nephites seems impossible. But perhaps that skepticism on the part of Mormons has as much to do with the loss of the Nephite-Mahdite experience of time as with anything else.

Citation Index

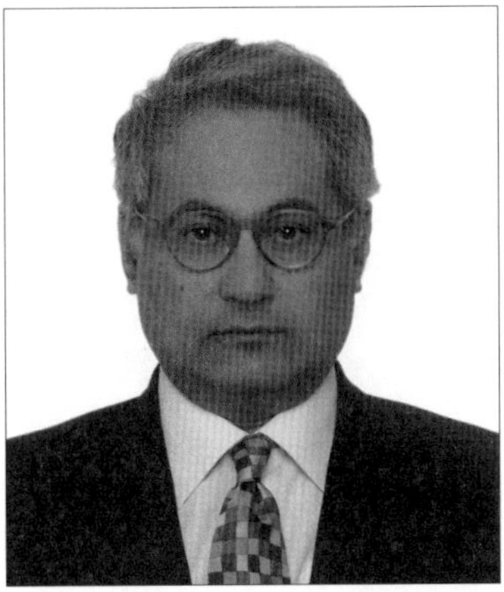

Jad Hatem is a professor of philosophy, literature, and religion at Saint Joseph University in Beirut, Lebanon, where he has taught since 1976. He has served as the chair of the philosophy department at the university, as also the director of the Centre d'études Michel Henry. He is the author of dozens of books. Among his most recent publications are *Qui est la vérité?* (Hermann, 2012), *L'Amour comme puissance et comme vérité* (Éditions du Cygne, 2012), and *Un bruit d'avoir été. Sur Qohélet* (Orizons, 2014).

About the Translator

Dr. Jonathon Penny is a published poet and scholar of letters whose work examines the intersection of theology and literature in surprising ways and places. He has taught at universities in the United States, Canada, and the Middle East.